THE CLINICAL PLACEMENT
A Nursing Survival Guide

D0761725

DEDICATIONS

This book is dedicated to my husband, Garry, and to my children, Joel, Ben, Cassie, Chelsea, Tyler and Madeline, for reminding me what matters most in life; and to my students, who continue to inspire me.
Tracy Levett-Jones

This book is a culmination of ideas, tested practices and experiences, and I would like to thank the many people who have contributed from multiple perspectives. Although I am unable to name these people who have inspired and worked with me, I would especially like to offer my special thanks to my husband, Patrice, who has been an undeniable tower of strength and support.
Sharon Bourgeois

Commissioning Editor: Ninette Premdas
Development Editors: Hannah Kenner, Janice Urquhart
Project Manager: Susan Stuart
Designer: George Ajayi

THE CLINICAL PLACEMENT
A Nursing Survival Guide

Tracy Levett-Jones
RN PhD MEd&Work BN DipAppSC(Nsg)

Deputy Head of School (Teaching and Learning)
Bachelor of Nursing Program Convenor and Senior Lecturer
School of Nursing and Midwifery
University of Newcastle, Australia

Sharon Bourgeois
RN PhD MEd MA BA FCN FRCNA

Associate Head of School and Senior Lecturer, School of Nursing and
Midwifery, University of Western Sydney, Australia

Consultant
Lynda Luke RM RN EN FPC BM BN

Public Health Staff Nurse, Family Planning Nurse and Midwife
Edinburgh, Developer and Administrator for
www.studentnurse.org.uk website and forum

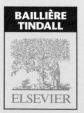

BAILLIÈRE TINDALL

ELSEVIER

Edinburgh   London   New York   Oxford   Philadelphia   St Louis   Sydney   Toronto   2009

BAILLIÈRE
TINDALL
ELSEVIER

© 2009, Elsevier Limited. All rights reserved.

First published © 2007 Elsevier, Australia

This book is adapted for Europe from the Australian edition published in 2007.

ISBN 978-0-7020-2970-7

British Library Cataloguing in Publication Data
A catalogue record for this book is available from the British Library

Library of Congress Cataloging in Publication Data
A catalog record for this book is available from the Library of Congress

Notice
Knowledge and best practice in this field are constantly changing. As new research and experience broaden our knowledge, changes in practice, treatment and drug therapy may become necessary or appropriate. Readers are advised to check the most current information provided (i) on procedures featured or (ii) by the manufacturer of each product to be administered, to verify the recommended dose or formula, the method and duration of administration, and contraindications. It is the responsibility of the practitioner, relying on their own experience and knowledge of the patient, to make diagnoses, to determine dosages and the best treatment for each individual patient, and to take all appropriate safety precautions. To the fullest extent of the law, neither the Publisher nor the Editors assume any liability for any injury and/or damage to persons or property arising out or related to any use of the material contained in this book.

The Publisher

Printed in China

Contents

Chapter 3   How you act   55

Chapter 4   How you think and feel   91

Chapter 5   How you communicate   115

Chapter 6   Insights from clinical experts   135

About the authors

Tracy Levett-Jones
RN PhD MEd&Work BN DipAppSC(Nsg)

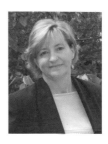

Tracy has a broad clinical and educational back-ground and has worked as a deputy head of school, director of clinical education, nurse educator, nurse manager, new graduate program coordinator and women's health nurse. Her research interests include clinical education, competency develop-ment and information and communication technology in healthcare.

Tracy believes that quality clinical placements are crucial to the development of capable and confident practitioners. Her doctoral studies explore the relationship between 'belonging' and the clinical experiences of nursing students in Australia and the United Kingdom. Tracy was the recipient of the 2007 New South Wales Minister for Education Quality Teaching Award.

Sharon Bourgeois
RN PhD MEd MA BA FCN FRCNA

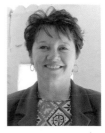

Sharon has been involved in several leadership roles associated with clinical education for nursing stu-dents including that of associate head of school and clinical director. She has also facilitated stu-dents' clinical and theoretical learning and sup-ported registered nurses' educational development. Her formal research interests have focused on the discourses of caring, and identifying 'an archive of caring for nursing'. Sharon has a strong interest in models of clinical education and the clinical learning environment and advocates that nurses embrace all elements of the professional role to enhance and promote care.

Preface

There is plenty of evidence, anecdotal and empirical, to suggest that clinical placements can be both tremendous and terrible. This book will help you to appreciate and capitalize on the tremendous, and to dodge or ride out the terrible, in what is sure to be one of the most exciting journeys of your life.

The aim of this book is to guide you on your clinical journey. It provides our shared viewpoints, based on many years of experience with students in clinical and academic settings. However, there are many other viewpoints, perspectives and opinions that are equally valid, and we encourage you to talk to academic and clinical staff, mentors, fellow students, friends and family about your placement experiences.

The ultimate goal of clinical education is the development of nurses who are confident and competent beginning practitioners. A positive and productive placement experience is pivotal to your success. This book encourages you to use your clinical placement as an opportunity to develop the skills and knowledge that under-pin quality practice, and to appreciate the clinical environment for the wonderful learning experience that it provides.

While deceptively simple, this book explores complex clinical learning issues. Although it is written primarily for nursing students, it will also be of interest to anyone involved in the clinical education of undergraduate students. Academics, clinicians, mentors and managers will find the information it contains useful as a stimulus for dialogue and debate. The book's interactive style and 'plain English' language approach are designed to engage with active readers and to encourage them to integrate the material into their practice.

How to use this book

Each chapter consists of a number of different sections. Within these sections, theory is interwoven to explain core principles. **Stories and scenarios** appear throughout the book to help you relate theory to the reality of practice. **Something to think about** boxes provide words of wisdom to reflect on and valuable snippets of advice. **Coaching tips** allow you to apply what you learn to your placement experiences.

The book is set out so that you can read from front to back. However, you may feel that some parts are more relevant to you than others, in which case you can simply skip back and forth.

Chapter 1 sets the scene by focusing on the 'rules of engagement' in complex clinical environments. The clinical context and culture are described and coaching tips provided to help you navigate your way successfully through this dynamic and exciting journey.

Chapter 2 provides insights into the 'great expectations' placed upon nursing students by patients, clinicians and the nursing profession as a whole. Armed with a clear understanding of what is required as you traverse the clinical learning milieu, your chances of success will be multiplied.

Chapter 3 gives a practical and positive description of how to behave and act within clinical environments. Tips for maximizing learning opportunities are provided, along with strategies for dealing with difficult and challenging situations.

Chapter 4 focuses on the beliefs, attitudes and values that underpin successful clinical performance, and encourages you to think about and reflect on your experiences in ways that are meaningful and relevant.

Chapter 5 looks at the ways nurses define and promote their profession through effective communication and gives advice on how to interact with clients and colleagues.

Chapter 6 is a compilation of sections written by expert nurses. We are delighted to include the viewpoints and perspectives of people from a wide cross-section of nursing specialties as they introduce you to the particular learning opportunities and challenges inherent in diverse clinical areas. Of course, we haven't been able to cover every clinical specialty, but we hope that the selection included opens your eyes to the wonderful opportunities available to nursing students and to graduates.

At the end of each chapter we have included **reflective thinking activities**. We encourage you to undertake these activities and to reflect carefully and critically about your ongoing progress as a nurse. Remember – nursing is a journey, not a destination.

We hope that you enjoy our book and that it helps you achieve success in your nursing journey.

Tracy Levett-Jones
Sharon Bourgeois

Chapter 1

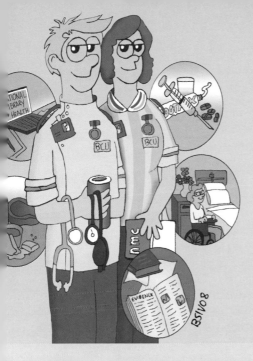

The rules of engagement

Always bear in mind that your own resolution to succeed is more important than any one thing.

Abraham Lincoln (1809–1865), 16th US president

Introduction

In this chapter we introduce you to the social world of nursing and the key people you will encounter on clinical placements. We attempt to make the 'implicit' explicit by sharing some of the hidden assumptions and understandings that underlie clinical practice and clinical cultures. In essence, this chapter will give you insight into what makes contemporary practice so complex, dynamic, challenging and very, very rewarding. It will help you to find your 'place' in clinical practice environments and equip you to work effectively with professional nurses and other health staff.

1.1 Know the lie of the land

The healthcare context has become increasingly complex, technological, consumer oriented and litigious over the last 20 years. Factors such as high patient throughput, increased acuity and decreased length of stay mean that hospitalized patients are sicker than ever before and stay in hospital for increasingly shorter periods of time. 'People admitted to general wards today were in intensive care fifteen years ago, many people cared for in hospital are now cared for in the community, and the people who are now in intensive care would have died fifteen years ago' (Johnson & Preston 2001, p 6). These factors, coupled with current nursing shortages, have made nurses' working lives challenging, intense and often stressful. In fact, the clinical learning environment may resemble a 'minefield for the unwary'.

Something to think about...

It was the best of times; it was the worst of times.
Charles Dickens (1812–1870), *A Tale of Two Cities*

Coaching tips

Why are we sharing this somewhat bleak outlook with you? Certainly not to discourage you from your chosen career path, but with the wisdom of knowing that 'forewarned is forearmed'. You'd be foolish to travel to a foreign land plagued by political and civil unrest without some degree of preparation in order to develop an understanding of the culture, people and context. The clinical learning environment is no different. Without an understanding of all that nursing in contemporary healthcare contexts means, you may well find yourself disillusioned by the dichotomy between what you *think* nurses and nursing should be and what they *actually* are.

Let's be very clear about one thing at this point: although the challenges associated with nursing in contemporary practice environments have escalated, the rewards, the satisfaction and the sheer joy in knowing you have made a difference are as wonderful today as they have always been. You will be inspired as you observe committed nurses providing extraordinary care despite, and perhaps even because of, the clinical challenges they encounter. Your mission (should you choose to accept it) is to navigate your way through what may seem at times to be a maze. This book will prepare you for your journey into this dynamic, exciting and challenging clinical environment.

Something to think about...

Travel plans are like honey, dripping down toward your lips – sweet anticipation.
Kurt Vonnegut (1922–2007), US novelist

1.2 The clinical placement – what it is and why it matters

Clinical placements (sometimes called clinical practicum, fieldwork or practice experiences) are where the world of nursing comes alive. At university or college you will learn *about nursing*. On your clinical placements you will learn *to nurse*. You will learn how nurses think, feel and behave, what they value and how they communicate. You will come to understand the culture and ethos of nursing in contemporary practice, as well as the problems, complexities and challenges nurses encounter. Some students say that clinical placements change the way they view the world. Whether this is true for you will depend to a large extent on how you approach it. Most importantly, clinical placements provide opportunities to engage with and care for clients, to enter their world, and to establish meaningful therapeutic relationships.

Clinical learning

Good nurses have a significant impact upon the clients and communities they serve. There is solid evidence (Aitken & Patrician 2000) that demonstrates that quality nursing care results in reductions in patient mortality and critical incidents such as medication errors, patient falls, hospital-acquired infections and pressure ulcers, to name a few. Clinical placements are where you apply the theory and knowledge gained through your academic pursuits to the reality of practice. Additionally, your clinical placement experiences will

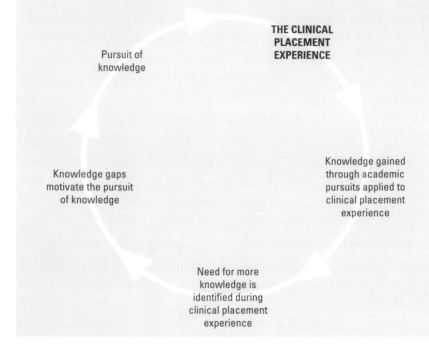

Figure 1.1   The cyclical nature of the pursuit of knowledge and clinical application.

make explicit the areas in which you need more knowledge and experience. In this way, the pursuit of knowledge and clinical application become an ongoing cycle of learning (Fig. 1.1).

Clinical placement experience structure and settings

In line with the European Union Directives (1977a,b), the Nursing and Midwifery Council (NMC 2002) has determined that nursing programmes are to be 4600 hours long and comprise 50% theory and 50% clinical practice learning. The purpose of these requirements is to achieve mutual recognition of formal nursing qualifications by all members of the European Union (EU), and to define the minimum standards to be observed by each member country.

In the UK there are three pre-registration award programmes: degree, diploma and advanced diploma. Nursing students complete a common foundation programme for 1 year and then pursue their choice of branch – adult, paediatric, learning disability or mental health nursing for the next 2 years. The NMC and the EU Directives prescribe the type of experience that students must have in order to be eligible for registration. Students in the adult nursing branch undertake clinical placements in a variety of facilities, including hospital wards, clinics and community settings such as nursing homes, visits to clients' homes and local health centres. Students enrolled in the mental health branch often gain experience in a range of mental health settings, as well as one general nursing placement aimed at developing physical nursing skills. Similarly, learning disability placements include a broad range of settings in addition to one placement in mainstream health services. Students studying in the field of children's nursing undertake placements across a range of settings aimed at learning about the healthy child and providing care for children and young children experiencing ill-health. Each of these specialty clinical areas has inherent learning opportunities and challenges. In Chapter 6, nursing experts from these practice areas share their insights. They provide an overview of each area, the unique learning opportunities available and the clinical challenges that you may encounter.

In most universities, clinical visits usually occur in first or second semester. Depending on where you study, the length of each place-ment experience will vary. Clinical shifts vary from 7.5 to 13 hours (called long days). Rotas are full time and may be organized by you in negotiation with your ward sister and/or mentor. You should expect to work the same shifts as your mentor for at least three out of five shifts per week. It is a good idea (and in fact some universi-ties require it) for you make an appointment to visit your mentor prior to beginning your practice experience. This will allow you to organize your rota, discuss your expectations and learning objectives, and generally orient yourself to the unit.

Clinical supervision and support

During your practice experiences you will have a mentor and/or a practice teacher to guide your learning and to support you. How-ever, it is important to remember that, to a large extent, the success of your placement will depend on what you bring to it and your degree of preparation and motivation.

Your feelings before, during and after your clinical placement experience will vary. Students report experiencing some or all of the following emotions: excitement, exhilaration, pride, confusion, anxiety, fear, apprehension, tension and stress. Your mentor or practice teacher is there to support you. It is important to share your feelings and to seek further guidance and support whenever necessary.

Coaching tips

- The first step in preparing for your journey into the clinical placement is to make sure you are familiar with your educational institution's guidelines, procedures, policies and contact people.
- The second step (of course) is to read this book!

What's in a name?

When describing the people nurses care for, this book is peppered with the terms patient, client, service user and resident. We made the decision to use these different terms deliberately. When you undertake clinical placements you will quickly become aware that different terms are used to refer to those you care for, depending on the context of practice. We define the terms here so that you'll have a clear understanding of their meaning.

Patient is still the most common term used to describe a person seeking or receiving health care. It does carry some negative connotations, however, as traditionally a 'patient' was defined as someone who passively endured pain or illness. Although patients are becoming more active and proactive where their health is concerned, the term 'patient' is still the one you'll hear most often.

Client refers to the recipient of nursing care. Client is a term that is inclusive of individuals, significant others, families and communities. It applies to people who are well and those who are experiencing health changes. It is intended to recognize the recipient of care as an active partner in that care, and the need for the nurse to engage in professional behaviours that facilitate this active partnership. The term 'client' is often used in mental health and community health services.

panel continues

What's in a name? (continued)

Resident most often refers to a person who resides in an aged care facility or a person with a developmental disability who lives in a residential care facility, either short or long term.

Service user is considered by some to be a politically correct term. In contemporary health care, service user is a term that is inclusive of consumers, clients, patients and carers. Service user involvement is defined as an active and equitable collaboration between professionals and clients concerning the planning, implementation and evaluation of health services. Implicit in this definition is the transfer of power or control over aspects of service delivery from professionals to clients (Wright & Rowe 2005). Thus, the term 'service user' denotes an active role in the planning and delivery of health services.

As you can see, there are divided opinions about the 'correct' terms to describe those we care for. We suggest that you keep an open mind during your clinical placements.

1.3 Patient-centred care

'Patient- or person-centred care' is a term that has become prevalent in the nursing literature over the past decade. It is a notion that nurses hold dear, particularly in the increasingly complex and busy environments typical of contemporary practice. You will hear this term used frequently, so it is important to understand its meaning and application in clinical practice.

Patient- or person-centred care has been defined by McCormack (2004) as being concerned with the authenticity of the individual, that is, their personhood. It is a way of working that focuses on patients' personal beliefs, values, wants, needs and desires. Person-centred practice requires nurses to know the values held by their patients in order to treat them as individuals. Patient-centred care adopts approaches that enable flexibility, mutuality, respect, care and being with another in an interconnected relationship (McCormack 2004). Within this approach, nurses must recognize patients' freedom to make their own decisions as a fundamental and valuable human right. Simply stated, patient-centred care means holistic care and placing people at the centre of all of the care decisions that are made.

Coaching tips

Consider the following situations.

A newly qualified nurse was practising her intravenous cannulation (an aseptic technique performed by medical or nursing staff to gain peripheral venous access in order to administer fluids, blood or medications) skills, as she required ten successful attempts to be accredited. Her patient, a 96-year-old woman, was admitted from an aged care facility with anaemia (a reduction in the number of red blood cells or the amount of haemoglobin in the blood), secondary to a long history of melaena (abnormally dark tarry faeces containing blood that is usually from gastrointestinal bleeding). The patient had expressed reluctance to have the blood transfusion that had been ordered for her. Despite the patient's obvious pain and distress, the nurse unsuccessfully attempted the cannulation four times, before giving up. She was dismissive of the patient's concerns about the transfusion.

Although it was important for this nurse to be re-accredited, was it more important than the patient's well-being? Was her care patient centred? In the competing priorities evident in this scenario, did the patient's needs and values take precedence?

In another situation, a student nurse wanted to learn how to perform a urinary catheterization. She entered the patient's room, explained that she was there to observe the catheterization, and proceeded to watch the registered nurse perform the procedure. She did not seek the patient's consent, nor was she aware of his discomfort and embarrassment resulting from her presence.

Once again the patient's feelings, needs and rights were not paramount. Even if the patient's verbal consent had been sought, the nurse should have paid careful attention to his verbal and non-verbal responses, such as facial expressions and body language, which may well have revealed a different story.

We've given two examples where patient-centred care was not evident. Now we share a story where the opposite was true.

Emma [pseudonym] was an 18-year-old woman admitted to a palliative care unit with terminal cancer. All of the nursing staff on the unit had become involved in her care, particularly the nurse in charge. When Emma realized that she would not be returning home, she became terribly despondent. The nurse spoke to her family and organized a secret 'rendezvous' in the hospital basement, at the service entrance. When Emma was wheeled down to the basement in her hospital bed, surrounded by infusion pumps, syringe drivers and other nursing paraphernalia, she was greeted by her adored Maltese terrier, Zoe. The look of absolute joy on Emma's face as Zoe snuggled into her arms for the last time was unforgettable.

This caring nurse's organization of a 'rendezvous' was a challenging feat, but it exemplifies perfectly what patient-centred care really means.

How nurses think, behave and speak should be underpinned by a commitment to patient-centred care. When caring for your patients reflect on whether your practice is patient-centred – our patients deserve nothing less.

1.4 Models of care

Undertaking clinical placements in different facilities and units will provide you with exposure to different models of patient care. A model of care provides a framework for the way that patient care is organized within an area of practice, and relates to the way that nurses and other healthcare workers within the team structure patient care activities. Differences in the models of care implemented within units or wards can be attributed to several factors, including the current worldwide shortage of nurses (Fagin 2001) and differences in skill mix (numbers, types and levels of experience of nurses and healthcare workers) (Davidson et al 2006; Hurst 2002; Viens et al 2005).

Throughout the world there have been major changes to how care is delivered (Holland et al 2008). Models of patient care may include:

- task-oriented nursing
- team nursing
- patient allocation, total patient care or case management.

Task-oriented nursing refers to a model whereby nurses undertake specific tasks related to nursing care across a group of patients. Some examples of task allocation may be when a nurse undertakes to shower all patients in a ward; another nurse may undertake the medications for the same group of patients. In this model of care delivery, nursing care relates to sets of activities that are performed by nurses for patients.

Team nursing is a model that 'teams' experienced permanent nurses with less experienced or casual staff to achieve nursing goals using a group approach. The size and skill mix of teams can vary from unit to unit and across healthcare facilities.

Patient allocation models were developed because nurses recognized the need for total patient care. The implementation of these types of model results in nurses getting to know the whole patient, rather than patients being cared for as a series of tasks. A nurse will be allocated to his or her patients (the number is dependent on factors such as patients' needs, staff mix and ward policies) and undertake all nursing care for the allocated patient.

The model of care delivery implemented on a ward will depend on a range of factors, including the degree of innovation and commitment by the people involved. Some models work better when there are sufficient numbers of highly qualified staff (registered nurse) to deliver care; others may focus on supporting less experienced staff using a team approach.

Activity

On your next placement, identify the model of care delivery used in the unit. Discuss with the nurses the reasons for the implementation of this model and its advantages and disadvantages. Find out where student nurses fit into this model.

1.5 Competent and proficient practice

Competence and proficiency are complex concepts that are difficult to define and measure (FitzGerald et al 2001). Many people make the mistake of thinking that being competent or proficient simply means that you can satisfactorily perform a set task, but competence and proficiency are so much more than this. Girot (1993, p 85) provides a more complete definition by suggesting 'the ability to combine knowledge, skills, behaviours, attitudes, values and beliefs appropriate to professional service delivery across a variety of contexts' is what truly determines a competent or proficient nurse.

The NMC has developed the standards of proficiency to describe the attributes and performance required of a proficient nurse in the clinical setting. These proficiencies provide a benchmark for assessment. You will need to become very familiar with these standards, as your fitness for practice will be assessed using these criteria (NMC 2004a).

Keep in mind that 'proficient' does not mean 'expert'. There are various levels of proficiency, but each of these has a minimum acceptable level or standard. Beginners are rarely expert, but they can be proficient at performing a wide range of nursing activities methodically and well. They may be slow, but in time beginners develop organizational and time-management skills. They ask many questions (as they should), but they know the right questions to ask.

What does it all mean?

Competence represents the overall ability of an individual to perform effectively within a role. This includes the knowledge, skills, attitudes and experience to undertake a whole role to the standard expected of like persons within a similar environment (Royal College of Nursing 2005).

Competency describes the skills and abilities to practise safely and effectively without the need for direct supervision. Competencies are achieved incrementally throughout periods of clinical placement experience during a programme. At the end of the final period of placement experience or supervised practice, it is the evidence of achievement of all competencies that enables sign-off by mentors or practice teachers (NMC 2006).

Practice proficiency Students are deemed proficient when they have successfully met all the NMC standards of proficiency for nursing, midwifery or specialist community public health nursing, or the relevant outcomes of a NMC specialist practice qualification, at the end of a NMC-approved programme. Practice proficiency may be signed off only by a practice teacher or a mentor who has met the additional NMC criteria (NMC 2005a).

Proficiencies These are contained within the standards of proficiency for each of the three parts of the register. Fitness for practice is demonstrated by meeting all NMC proficiencies and other requirements by the end of the programme (NMC 2005a).

Coaching tips

The last decade has seen a plethora of reports that highlight problems related to the development and demonstration of clinical proficiency by newly qualified nurses (Council of Deans and Heads of UK University Faculties for Nursing Midwifery and Health Visiting 1998; Department of Health 1999, 2000; Peach 1999). In these coaching tips we suggest ways of developing your proficiency during your studies and throughout your nursing career.

Be knowledgeable
- Focus on understanding the concepts and principles that underpin nursing care. Knowing why is just as important as knowing how.
- Ask questions, read widely, think carefully.
- Develop your library skills so that you can find the best information fast.
- Develop your research skills so that you can discern what is good, better and the best evidence for practice.
- When on a clinical placement attend in-service training whenever you have the opportunity.
- Find out when conferences are being held that are relevant to your learning and attend if possible – they are a great way of networking and accessing cutting-edge information.
- Aim high in your academic pursuits – don't be content with 'just a pass'.
- Attend all of your lectures and tutorials on campus (don't skip classes).
- Commit to becoming a self-directed, lifelong learner. Remember, 'Knowledge keeps no better than fish' (Burnard & Chapman 1990, p 11) and, given the rapid scientific and technological advances in the healthcare field, the knowledge gained in your programme of study may soon become obsolete.

Develop your skills
- Work hard to develop your skills – attend all clinical skills sessions and participate actively.
- Don't miss an opportunity to practise. Many educational institutions encourage students to practise outside scheduled classes. These are valuable opportunities to consolidate your skills and identify any weaknesses.

- Observe expert clinicians caring for their patients. Ask them to supervise and critique your practice.
- There are many types of clinical skill checklist available and they are excellent for assessment purposes. Students can peer-review one another, and your mentor may use them to assess you as well. In some programmes the assessment of core skills using a designated checklist is a compulsory requirement.
- Continually ask yourself, 'Is my practice safe and effective, and am I adhering to the principles of best practice?'.

Reflect on your behaviours, values, attitudes and beliefs
- Nursing is a process of personal and professional growth. Throughout your studies, and indeed your career, it is vitally important to consider and reconsider your values, attitudes and beliefs continually, and to analyse how these attributes are reflected in your behaviours.
- Reflect on what it is that you value most – in yourself and in other professionals. Is it honesty, integrity, work ethic, compassion? Then consider how these values can be developed and integrated into your practice.
- Challenge your preconceptions. Listen and be open to other people's perspectives, particularly if their opinions are different from yours.
- Immerse yourself in a wide range of literature and media that challenge your thinking and the way you view the world.
- There are few worse criticisms for a nurse than to be called narrow minded or bigoted.
- Embrace cultural diversity and open your mind (and heart) to people with different ethnicity, nationality, religion, language, age, gender and lifestyle – listen and learn!

1.6 Working within your scope of practice

The professional conduct of a registered nurse, midwife or specialist community public health nurse is governed by the NMC code of professional conduct. It is this code that students of nursing strive to meet within their practice also. Nursing programmes differ significantly, so students' practice will vary depending on where they are studying. Your practice will develop as your level of proficiency increases, and may vary depending on the context of your placement.

Consider the following situation.

A first-year student was concerned and upset about his unsatisfactory clinical result. He felt discouraged because he was a high-achieving student and expected that he would meet all requirements easily. His mentor had written the following comment: 'Casmir is a hardworking and committed student but needs to work within the code of professional conduct and focus on consolidating skills appropriate to his educational level'.

When asked to describe his practice experience and what had prompted this comment from the mentor, Casmir explained that he'd had a great placement, and had been given wonderful learning opportunities by the registered nurses on his ward. He'd been permitted to do central line dressings, titrate intravenous (IV) infusions, manage patient-controlled analgesia (PCA), and more. He was proud that he had learnt skills well beyond those of most first-year students and was annoyed that the mentor did not applaud his initiative.

Casmir had little understanding of the purpose or potential complications of central lines, infusion pumps or PCA, and had been so focused on these advanced skills that he'd had little time to practise and consolidate skills more appropriate to his level of education. He was not confident with patient hygiene, nor was he able to administer oral medications safely even when supervised by his mentor. Casmir was trying to run before he could walk.

Casmir had practised nursing skills beyond his level of knowledge and therefore was unsafe. Although the code of professional conduct and standards for conduct, performance and ethics (NMC 2004b) is not intended to limit learning opportunities, it does provide a framework for practice.

Why do you need to discuss with the nurses you work with the nursing activities that are appropriate for you to undertake?

Clinicians frequently express the concern that they are not clear about what students have learnt on campus and in previous placement experiences. Additionally, they are unsure of what clinical activities students should be encouraged to engage in during practice experiences. Clinicians often describe instances where students attempt procedural skills beyond their level of ability, or alternatively are reluctant to engage in clinical experiences outside their 'comfort zone'. A clear and agreed upon understanding of the nursing skills students can undertake will allow clinicians to support and challenge students based upon a collaborative understanding of expectations.

Coaching tips

- Make sure you access and understand the NMC code of professional conduct (NMC 2008) and undertake practice appropriate to your university/college guidelines.
- Clarify your university/college instructions for practice. Some educational institutions will not permit you to attempt any nursing procedures that: (a) are not explicitly identified in a clinical practice document, or (b) students have not practised or demonstrated proficiency in. Be aware that different institutions have different requirements.
- Share your ideas about practice opportunities with your mentor and the nurses you work with, so that they know how they can best support and guide you.
- When asked to perform beyond your level of experience and learning, simply explain your institution's guidelines. Of course you'll express your interest and say that you'd really like to watch the procedure being performed by an expert nurse.

1.7 To whom shall I turn?

During your clinical placements, supportive relationships with nursing colleagues have the potential to ease the transition between the relatively sheltered world of academia and the health service environment, with all its contemporary challenges and pressures.

Coaching tips

Irrespective of whether you are supported by a mentor, a practice teacher or other clinical staff, to a large extent the success of these relationships will depend on you. You need to be very clear about your learning objectives (see Section 3.12), as these will frame your learning, and you must be able to explain them so that the person you are working with can support you and guide you towards achieving them. Occasionally, if your objectives are not achievable or appropriate for a particular environment, your mentor may suggest that they need to be modified or amended.

You will probably find that your mentor will observe and assess you for a while before entrusting you with independent patient care. Don't take this personally or as an indication of a lack of confidence in your ability. It is only to be expected; registered nurses maintain responsibility for their patients at all times and your mentor will want to be very sure of your abilities before allowing you to practise with any measure of independence.

If a situation arises in which you feel that your relationship with your mentor is not working, try to resolve it with him or her in the first instance. Be open to his or her viewpoints, as it may just be a problem of miscommunication. However, if this does not improve the situation or if you feel uncomfortable about trying to resolve it, you should seek the support and guidance of someone experienced whom you feel you can trust to handle the situation professionally – your academic support person (e.g. link lecturer) may be ideal.

Nursing mirrors what happens in everyday life and sometimes personality clashes arise. Hopefully these can be managed in a positive, professional and constructive manner, but at times it may be best for you to work with a different mentor. Be mindful that experiencing a series of personality clashes may indicate that you need some guidance in managing interpersonal relationships.

To whom shall I turn?

Mentor Traditionally, mentoring referred to a mutual and committed relationship between a student and an experienced staff member. The relationship developed over time and created opportunities for students to gain valuable skills and knowledge, to become socialized and acculturated to the organization and its ways of operating, and to become proficient in the new role under the direct guidance of the mentor. Mentors should be experienced nurses who have undertaken mentorship training or have an equivalent qualification in their own field.

The main responsibilities of the mentor include:

- supervision of a student's performance and behaviour while on placement
- formative and summative assessment of practice competencies to ensure that the student meets the NMC standards for pre-qualifying programmes
- liaison with designated university staff if there is an issue that may be affecting the student's progress.

panel continues

To whom shall I turn? (continued)

Sign-off mentor A mentor who has met specified criteria (outcomes of stage 2) in order to be able to sign off a student's practice proficiency at the end of a NMC approved programme.

Practice teacher (or lecturer practitioner) A registered nurse who has gained knowledge, skills and competence both in a specialist area of practice and in a teaching role. Practice teachers facilitate student learning, and supervise and assess students in the practice setting. They will have undertaken a NMC approved teacher preparation programme, or equivalent, and successfully achieved the outcomes defined in stage 4 of the developmental framework.

Link lecturer Link lecturers are responsible for liaising with clinical staff to monitor the quality of practice experiences. They offer support to students and registered nurses as well as advise students and staff on educational matters.

Learning environment facilitators (or practice education facilitators) Registered nurses who are based in NHS Trusts and the independent sector to support mentors and manage practice-based learning issues. Their main responsibilities include:

- developing and supporting the quality of learning experiences and learning opportunities
- developing the mentors and other staff with whom students will be working
- working in partnership with practitioners, students, the university/college, the NHS and the independent sector to manage practice-based learning issues
- supporting mentors in developing innovative ways of learning and sharing good practice
- ensuring practice experiences enable students to meet learning outcomes of the award that they are enrolled in by developing fitness for practice within the nursing profession.

(NMC 2005a, 2006; Royal College of Nursing 2005):

Something to think about...

Mentors remind us that we can indeed survive the terror of the coming journey and undergo the transformation by moving through, not around our fear. Mentors give us the magic that allows us to enter the darkness, a talisman to protect us from evil spells, a gem of wise advice, a map, and sometimes simply courage. But always the mentor appears near the onset of the journey as a helper, equipping us in some way for what is to come, a midwife to our dreams, a 'keeper of the promise'. Success is a lot slipperier without a mentor to show us the ropes. The mentor is clearly concerned with the transmission of wisdom. They do this by leading us on the journey of our lives. We trust them because they have been there before. They embody our hopes, cast light on the way ahead, interpret arcane signs, warn us of lurking dangers, and point out unexpected delights along the way.

Daloz (1999, p 18)

1.8 Working hard – but not too hard

Nursing students frequently express how important it is for them to fit in – to belong and be accepted as part of the nursing team. This is not surprising, given that the need to belong has been cited as a fundamental human need (Baumeister & Leary 1995; Maslow 1987). Students who try too hard to fit in sometimes sacrifice their 'student status' to become one of the 'workers'. It is not unusual for students, believing that their hard work will help them to be valued as part of the team, to fill their clinical placement days with a series of disjointed nursing tasks (making beds, taking vital signs, bathing patients), rather than developing their ability to nurse holistically. Don't be confused! We are not saying that students are above basic nursing skills. On the contrary, we are saying that as a student you need to be proactive in identifying and maximizing valuable learning opportunities across a range of areas and at different levels.

Something to think about...

When a child stands in awe of the mystery of a falling rose petal, then it's time to teach the law of gravity.

Anonymous

Coaching tips

Give yourself permission to be a student! Articulate your learning objectives and assessment requirements. Be on the lookout for serendipitous learning opportunities. Listen closely in handover and relate your clinical objectives to the clinical issues identified. Did someone mention a complex diabetic leg ulcer that needs to be re-dressed? Do you have wound management as one of your objectives? Take the initiative. Ask if you can watch the wound dressing being performed, then go home that night and read all you can about diabetic ulcers. The next day ask if you can undertake the procedure under supervision. As a student it is your responsibility to link theory and practice, and you will have countless opportunities to do so (if you are on the lookout for them). Linking theory to practice will allow you to develop your repertoire of knowledge and skills in a way that is clinically relevant.

Ask whether you can care for increasing numbers of patients (under supervision), so that you can develop your time-management and organizational skills (even in first year). Certainly, while caring for groups of patients you'll be doing so-called 'basic skills' (never forget how important they are and how much consolidation they need), but you'll also be extending your practice and learning to nurse holistically rather than in a task-oriented way.

Don't fool yourself into thinking that if you just 'get on with the job' you'll fit in and be accepted. You are much more likely to earn the respect of your clinical colleagues by fully embracing your student status, asking questions, seeking out learning opportunities and showing an interest.

1.9 Privacy

Several pieces of government legislation require the protection of personal information and the privacy of others. This type of legislation ensures that information about individuals is not used without their consent or for illegal purposes. Privacy is a right for all individuals and you will need to ensure that you understand your obligations with respect to data protection, access to health records and freedom of information (Department of Health 2007; Ministry of Justice 2007a; NMC 2007).

You are obliged to protect and maintain personal information about others during the course of clinical placement. You should understand your patients' wishes with regard to the sharing of information with their family or others. Likewise, this requirement applies to you, and you can also expect that your personal information is protected. Personal information is information that can identify someone. This could include your name, address or phone number. Health information (for example, health records) is also protected (Department of Health 2007; Ministry of Justice 2007b; NMC 2007).

Information about individuals must not be used illegally or given to others without the individual's consent. Most educational institutions will have processes available for students to lodge concerns if they feel that their privacy has been breached. Health facilities also have these mechanisms available to patients and staff. You need to take care to ensure that you do not inadvertently disclose client information. Some areas where you will need to be particularly mindful include the notes you take during handover and any discussions you are involved in, including debriefing sessions.

Aside from considering patient privacy concerns, on clinical placements you will be exposed to issues that may affect other students. Be prudent in your behaviours, to ensure that incidents that occur with fellow students during placements are not relayed to other students on campus. The following story relates an example that occurred recently.

Mary was on the same ward as André for their second-year placement. During the last few days of the placement, André had been arguing with his mentor about what he believed he should be doing. The mentor had pointed out that André was to care for his allocated patients to the level of his knowledge and was not on placement just to undertake clinical assessments. André was instructed to negotiate his learning with clinical staff, as well as to take responsibility for the care of his patients. Over the course of the placement, several staff had complained to the mentor about André's lack of patient care. The mentor discussed the issues and strategies for improvement with André, but following a lack of improvement he eventually received an unsatisfactory grade for his placement.

On return to university the following week, André was angry when several students spoke to him about his unsatisfactory clinical report. André confronted Mary about how other students had become aware of his clinical result and her role in disclosing information about his placement.

In this scenario, Mary had revealed private information about André. While she had not mentioned his name, the other students were able to identify him from the situation as it had been described.

Remember, the privacy of individuals and personal information is protected by government legislation and in all situations you must protect the personal information of others.

Coaching tips

- Be aware of what constitutes privacy and breaches of privacy, and the laws related to these issues.
- Protect information about a person whose identity is apparent or whose identity can be reasonably ascertained from information provided.
- Access to any information about patients, including patients' notes, requires permission.
- Gain consent to use potentially identifiable information (written consent is preferable). Some circumstances may require the medical officer and the sister in charge to give consent.
- Remember, individuals have the right to control their own personal information, and valid consent must be obtained prior to the use of that information.
- Collect only the minimum amount of information about a person after obtaining his or her consent.
- Seek advice and guidance from management about policies and protocols in operation at every facility where you are placed. These will vary depending on the type of facility, its guiding policies and your health department directives.

1.10 Confidentiality

Something to think about...

Responsibility for sensitive confidential information about clients or patients is often both a burden and a privilege for carers, but it also gives them a special relationship with those in their care and subtle power over them.

Thompson et al (2000, p 119)

Confidentiality can be defined as a professional obligation to respect privileged information between health provider and client. Consider the following situation.

Joseph was sitting at the coffee shop when some of his fellow students wandered in to join him. They were excited about having witnessed the birth of a baby and wanted to share their experiences. However, Joseph became uncomfortable when one of his colleagues began to speak explicitly about the delivery, complications that had occurred and even mentioned the name the parents had given their new baby. Joseph cautioned his colleagues about maintaining confidentiality and requested that they keep their voices low, so that people nearby could not hear. Although his colleagues were initially annoyed about being criticized and felt somewhat belittled by Joseph's comments, they soon complied.

People often disclose sensitive and sometimes private information about themselves to health professionals. However, in doing so, patients make themselves vulnerable (Thompson et al 2000). Safeguards to protect this vulnerability of patients are nested within the concept of confidentiality.

Confidentiality is a broad concept that extends the concept of privacy. Although nurses may discuss personal details and care related to patients, this discussion should be constrained by ethical standards and responsible judgement. The NMC code of professional conduct (NMC 2008) determines that nurses must protect confidential information.

Coaching tips

- Do not use patients' experiences as 'conversation pieces'. Disclosing bits of information may assist a listener to identify a person and therefore breaches confidentiality. Confidentiality means that you need to consider how information is used, handled, stored or restricted.
- Be aware of how you document handover notes and how these are used and safeguarded throughout your shift and following your shift.
- Ensure that you are familiar with policies and protocols in operation at healthcare facilities. These vary according to the type of facility and governmental policies, and include information used for assignment preparation. Use of client's notes and photographs will need to comply with the facility's protocols.

1.11 First impressions last

It's a sad but true fact that first impressions are formed within seconds of meeting and those impressions are based most often on appearance. Forget what you see on television. In the real world of nursing, a very specific dress code exists. The clinical environment is focused on safety – yours and that of the patients – and this to a large extent dictates what is considered acceptable in appearances in general, and uniforms in particular.

Don't be caught unaware – before you start your placement, check your educational institution's requirements as well as those of your placement venue. Some placements have special requirements; for example, mental health facilities may prefer smart casual clothes, whereas operating theatres usually provide surgical attire.

Below we offer some guidelines based on our experiences of what most clinical venues expect. We tried to find a way of writing this section that was discreet and delicate, but eventually decided just to 'say it like it is'!

Coaching tips

- Uniforms should be neat, complete, comfortable, correctly fitting, clean and wrinkle free.

- Shoes must be comfortable (for obvious reasons) and comply with occupational health and safety standards (non-slip, fully enclosed, leather).
- Heavy make-up is not appropriate for clinical placement – it is best left for your leisure time. Overpowering perfumes should be avoided, as they can cause patients to become nauseated.
- Nails should be clean, short, filed and without nail polish for infection control purposes. It is easy to tear the fragile skins of elderly patients or to penetrate gloves with long or sharp nails. Chipped nail polish and artificial nails have been shown to harbour infectious microorganisms.
- Long hair must be clean and tied back firmly above the collar.
- Leave your jewellery at home. Wristwatches are problematic as they can scratch patients and need to be removed each time you wash your hands. A fob watch with a second hand is more convenient. Similarly, rings can scratch patients and cause cross-infection. A plain band is acceptable in most clinical areas. One pair of small studs (in ears only) may be accepted, but bracelets or necklaces are not to be worn (unless of the medic alert type). Many a confused person has pulled or grabbed at a dangling necklace or earring (ouch!).
- For placements where smart casual clothing is requested in lieu of uniform, avoid wearing revealing clothing.
- Last but not least, make sure you always wear your ID or name badge and have your personal protective equipment (for example, safety glasses) with you on clinical placements.

1.12 Competing needs

A supportive clinical learning environment is viewed as essential to maximizing students' readiness for practice (Clare et al 2003). The very nature of the clinical placement, can however, create competition between the educational needs of students and the service needs of the facility. Students enter an environment where financial constraints, technology, the pace of change and staff mix can impact on optimal clinical learning experiences.

Some clinical placements can create a situation where the fulfilment of your personal learning needs may compete with service needs. An example would be when you are allocated a patient load but the needs of your allocated patients do not align with your clinical objectives. You may be required to care for patients with completely different conditions from those that you had hoped to focus on, and therefore your ability to meet your goals is substantially reduced. In another situation, the educational institution requirements may be incongruent with the clinical practice model implemented, for example when the unit uses a model of team nursing and the student expects to care holistically for a group of patients.

Coaching tips

- Develop an understanding of the different clinical practice models used in the clinical environment.
- Negotiate your learning needs with your mentor early in the placement. Do not leave this to the last day.
- Openly discuss any concerns that you have with competing needs as soon as they become apparent and, with your mentor, identify strategies to address them.

1.13 The generation gap

In the UK there is a gradually ageing workforce, with 60% of the nursing workforce older than 40 years and more than one in four older than 50 years (NMC 2005b). This means that in the nursing profession there is, and will continue to be, a wide generational cross-section. So let's think about nursing generations, and where you fit in.

A generation is an aggregate of people who share birth years, a common location in history and a collective persona. In nursing there may be up to three generations of nurses working together in one clinical area. Each generation has its own set of expectations, values, goals and motivators, and it is almost inevitable that there will be some clashes due to a lack of mutual understanding. Below we describe some of the attributes of the different generations that you may encounter on a clinical placement.

Generational diversity

Baby boomers (born 1941–60)
Baby boomers constitute the largest generation and are said to be characterized by rebellion in their youth and conservatism in their thirties, forties and beyond. They share the common traits of

ambition, loyalty and optimism. They are highly committed to their employer, often regarded as workaholics and reluctant to change jobs.

Generation X (born 1961–81)
While career advancement and personal development are key to this generation's happiness, they are constantly trying to balance career, family and leisure activities. They tend to be sceptical, competitive, autonomous, image conscious and in need of regular feedback about their performance. They value fun and humour in the workplace and are open to new job opportunities.

Generation Y (born 1981 onwards)
Members of this generation are highly aware of their rights and have a perception of workplace entitlement. They expect their employers to be flexible and to accommodate individual needs. They want to be continually learning and challenged, and are perceived to have short attention spans. They are conversant with technology. They are altruistic, ambitious and independent workers, who are socially and environmentally responsible. They see job and career change as inevitable.

What generation X thinks of baby boomers
- They are workaholics.
- They are self-righteous.
- They thrive on work-related politics.
- They demand constant validation.
- They need to lighten up – it's only a job!
- They are set in their ways.
- They have quit learning and are stuck in a rut – 'This is the way we've always done it!'.
- They are not technologically competent.
- They are cynical and pessimistic – 'I knew this would happen'.
- They need to get along with people and be liked.

What baby boomers think of generation X
- They are lazy.
- They are whingers.
- They spend too much time on the internet and email.
- They are self-focused.
- They are demanding and refuse to wait their turn.

- They have no work ethic.
- They are not loyal.
- They don't show respect.
- They arcn't committed.
- They have a 'you owe me' attitude.
- They are easily bored.

What generation X and baby boomers think of generation Y
- They are too competitive.
- They are more focused on learning and less on getting the work done.
- They are obsessed with information technology.
- They are aloof and tolerate teamwork only when absolutely necessary.
- They need supervision, guidance, support and mentoring.

(Adapted from Kupperschmidt 1998, 2001; Weston 2001)

Coaching tips

- To which generation do you belong? Think about the extent to which the attributes described apply to you.
- Next time you undertake a clinical placement, consider the different generations that constitute the nursing team.
- Be aware that the different generational attitudes towards work, learning, technology, feedback and teamwork are likely to result in misunderstandings at times, and try not to take it personally. Remember 'understanding breeds tolerance'.

1.14 Roles and functions of the multidisciplinary healthcare team

Efficient workplace practices come about by understanding and appreciating the diverse skills and expertise of the different members of the multidisciplinary healthcare team.

Aside from nurses, the multidisciplinary healthcare team may include medical and allied health personnel, pharmacists, pathologists, psychologists, counsellors, radiologists, occupational therapists and speech pathologists, to name a few. Table 1.1 identifies some of the different people you may encounter on a clinical placement.

Table 1.1 People you may encounter on a clinical placement

Role	Definition
Students – nursing and midwifery	People who are enrolled in educational programmes accredited by registration boards that authorize nursing. These may include undergraduate nurses and student midwives.
Registered nurse (RN)	A person whose name is recorded on the Nursing and Midwifery Council (NMC) register is entitled to call themselves a 'Registered nurse'. A first and second level of registered nurse is noted on the NMC register. The register identifies the field in which a nurse has gained proficiency, for example adult, mental health, learning disability or child nursing. More than one area of proficiency may be noted if additional study has been undertaken. All registered nurses are personally accountable for their own practice, and must practise within their requisite knowledge and skills.
Midwife	A person whose name is recorded on the register of midwives and whose practice is governed by standards set down by the NMC. A midwife works in partnership with women and their families to give care during pregnancy, labour and during the postnatal period. Opportunities in midwifery include working in healthcare systems and in private practice.
Specialist community public health nurse	A NMC-registered nurse who works with individuals, families and communities promoting health and preventing ill-health. These nurses work across disciplines and professions in collaborative partnerships to influence health of populations. The NMC identifies standards of proficiency and education for specialist community public health nursing education programmes.
Healthcare assistants (HCAs)	Various roles and duties are undertaken by healthcare assistants. These roles are bound by job descriptions that outline the level of accountability required for practice. HCAs may function independently or in collaboration with the multidisciplinary healthcare team.

table continues

Table 1.1   People you may encounter on a clinical placement—Cont'd

Role	Definition
Technicians	Various technical positions abound in healthcare facilities. Some of these have replaced nursing roles and others have supplementary roles in the care of clients. Examples of technical staff are technicians who work with specialist equipment, for example medical equipment technicians and sterile-supply technicians.
Medical personnel	You will encounter several levels of medical personnel during placement. Within the UK Health Service doctors are registered in order to take up a consultant posting. The medical personnel encountered will depend on the health care context and supervision available. Doctors you may meet in the UK Health Service include: • Medical students • Junior doctors (foundation year 1 and 2) • House officers • Registrars • General medical practitioners • Locums • Consultants (surgeons and physicians), in public or private facilities. Resident medical officers usually encountered in public hospitals include the following: • Intern • Resident medical officer (year 1–4) • Registrar (year 1–4) • Senior registrar. Consultant medical officers may have a position related to a medical specialty, such as the following positions: anaesthetists, surgeons, obstetricians, gynaecologists, physicians, pathologists, psychiatrists.
Psychologists	People who are engaged in the scientific study of the mind and behaviour, and may assist through clinical treatment and teaching. They may be concerned with different areas such

table continues

Table 1.1   People you may encounter on a clinical placement—Cont'd

Role	Definition
	as sport and exercise, education, and occupational or clinical psychology.
Podiatrist	Practitioners of podiatry (chiropody) who deal with the treatment of feet and their ailments.
Occupational therapist	People who employ a form of therapy for those recuperating from physical or mental disease or injury. They encourage rehabilitation through performance of the activities of daily living (such as washing and dressing, hobbies, crafts).
Speech therapists	People concerned with the study and treatment of clients with speech, communication, language and swallowing problems.
Counsellors	People who provide support through 'talking therapy' to patients and service users in many areas of health care.

Based on Baron & Kalsher 2002; Concise Medical Dictionary (Oxford Reference Online: http://www.oxfordreference.com/pub/views/home.html); General Medical Council 2007a,b; NHS Careers 2007; Nursing and Midwifery Council website (http://www.nmc-uk.org).

Coaching tips

- Attend multidisciplinary healthcare team meetings when possible.
- Become familiar with the roles and functions of all staff encountered on each clinical placement.
- Develop an understanding of how team members communicate and work collaboratively to provide quality care.

1.15 Networking

Nursing is all about building and maintaining relationships – in business this is called networking. Clinical placements provide wonderful opportunities for students to meet new people and to develop strong networks. Nurturing professional relationships is a mechanism that students should develop during their course, as it has the potential to open many doors. Establishing your network is a powerful strategy to achieve career goals.

Networking is about capitalizing on the multiple relationships that you will develop as a student. The process begins by thinking of the people who share your interests and values, and who could be helpful to you now and in the future: fellow students, academic staff, clinical experts, mentors or sisters, for example. The people you network with may be those from whom you need help or advice. They may also be those who require your help or advice. You may be surprised how far the 'ripples' of networking extend.

I remember Joaquin, a cleaner who worked on the first ward I worked on as a registered nurse. He had recently migrated from South America. Joaquin was a tireless worker and always ready to help. He related well to staff and patients alike. As we were both new to the unit, a camaraderie developed between us. He was studying to become a nurse and I gave him some nursing texts. Our lives soon diverged but 5 years later I met Joaquin again at an interview. He was then in charge of the unit to which I'd applied for a position as a staff nurse.

Coaching tips

- List the people in your current network, and then list the people you'd like to network with in the future. Think about the type of people who could help you achieve your career goals and those who may benefit from your help.
- Don't be afraid to ask for the help or advice you need (most people love to be needed).
- Reach out to others who may need your help and advice, such as new students and international students.
- If you meet a registered nurse who particularly inspires you, ask if she or he would agree to act as a professional mentor throughout your programme.
- Ask whether there is a mechanism for you to apply for employment (as a healthcare worker for example) on wards that you particularly enjoyed, or whether you can return for another placement at a later date.
- Join professional nursing groups (many have student rates) to develop networks and relationships.
- Be open to the opportunities available for your graduate employment and make the most of the networking prospects.

Reflective thinking activities

Think about what motivated you to become a nurse and what you expected nursing to be like.

_____

_____

_____

Have your experiences been different from what you initially expected? In what ways have your nursing experiences exceeded your expectations? Are there any ways in which nursing has disappointed you?

_____

_____

_____

How can you ensure that you achieve your learning objectives in clinical environments even when the staff are busy and the area is short-staffed?

_____

_____

_____

What do you think are your most important rights and responsibilities as a nursing student?

_____

_____

_____

References

Aitken L, Patrician P 2000 Measuring organizational traits of hospitals: the revised nursing work index. Nursing Research 49(3):146–153

Baron R A, Kalsher M J 2002 Essentials of psychology. Allyn & Bacon, Boston

Baumeister R, Leary M 1995 The need to belong: desire for interpersonal attachments as a fundamental human motivation. Psychological Bulletin 117(3):497–529

Burnard P, Chapman C 1990 Nurse education: the way forward. Scutari Press, Harrow

Clare J, Brown D, Edwards H et al 2003 Evaluating clinical learning environments: creating education–practice partnerships and clinical education benchmarks for nursing. Learning outcomes and curriculum development in major disciplines: nursing phase 2 final report, March. School of Nursing and Midwifery, Flinders University, Adelaide

Council of Deans and Heads of UK University Faculties for Nursing Midwifery and Health Visiting 1998 Breaking the boundaries: educating nurses, midwives and health visitors for the Next Millennium: a position paper.

Daloz N 1999 Guiding the journey of adult learners. Jossey Bass, San Francisco

Davidson P, Halcomb E, Hickman L et al 2006 Beyond rhetoric: what do we mean by a 'model of care'? Australian Journal of Advanced Nursing 23(3):47–55

Department of Health 1999 Making a difference. Strengthening the nursing, midwifery and health visiting contribution to health and healthcare. Department of Health, London

Department of Health 2000 The NHS plan. Department of Health, London

Department of Health 2007 Privacy policy. Online. Available: http://www. dh.gov.uk/en/DH_4110944 13 Aug 2007

European Union 1977a Directive 77/452/EEC. Online. Available: http:// euro-pa.eu.int/eur-lex/lex/LexUriServ.do?uri=CELEX:31977L0452:EN: HTML 20 Jun 2006

European Union 1977b Directive 77/453/EEC. Online. Available: http:// euro-pa.eu.int/eur-lex/lex/LexUriServ.do?uri=CELEX:31977L0453:EN: HTML 20 Jun 2006

Fagin C M 2001 When care becomes a burden: diminishing access to adequate nursing. Online. Available: http://www.milbank.org/010216fagin. html 23 Apr 2001

FitzGerald M, Walsh K, McCutcheon H 2001 An integrative systematic review of indicators for competence for practice and protocol for validation of indicators of competence. Conducted by the Joanna Briggs Institute for Evidence Based Nursing and Midwifery. Commissioned by the Queensland Nursing Council. Adelaide University, Adelaide

General Medical Council 2007a New registration framework for doctors. What it means for the registration of international medical students. Online. Available: http://www.gmc-uk.org/register/employing/ NRF_Final.pdf 13 Aug 2007

General Medical Council 2007b Education. Online. Available: http://www. gmc-uk.org/education/index.asp 13 Aug 2007

Girot E 1993 Assessment of competence in clinical practice: a review of the literature. Nurse Education Today 13:83–90

Holland K, Jenkins J, Solomon J, Whittam S (eds) 2008 Applying the Roper–Logan–Tierney model in practice. Churchill Livingstone, Elsevier, Edinburgh

Hurst K 2002 Selecting and applying methods for estimating the size and mix of nursing teams. A systematic review of the literature commissioned by the Department of Health. University of Leeds Nuffield Institute for Health, Leeds.

Johnson D, Preston B 2001 Australia: an overview of issues in nursing education. Online. Available: http://www.detya.gov.au/highered/eippubs/eip01_12fullreport.htm 30 Apr 2005

Kupperschmidt B 1998 Understanding generation X employees. Journal of Nursing Administration 28(12):36–43

Kupperschmidt B 2001 Understanding next generation employees. Journal of Nursing Administration 31(12):570–574

Maslow A 1987 Motivation and personality, 3rd edn. Harper & Row, New York

McCormack B 2004 Person-centredness in gerontological nursing: an overview of the literature. International Journal of Older People Nursing 13(3a):31–38

Ministry of Justice 2007a Data sharing and protection. Online. Available: http://www.justice.gov.uk/whatwedo/datasharingandprotection.htm 28 Feb 2008

Ministry of Justice 2007b Freedom of information. Online. Available: http://www.justice.gov.uk/whatwedo/freedomofinformation.htm 13 Aug 2007

NHS Careers 2007 Online. Available: http://www.nhscareers.nhs.uk 13 Aug 2007

Nursing and Midwifery Council 2002 Requirements for pre-registration nursing programmes. NMC, London

Nursing and Midwifery Council 2004a Standards of proficiency for pre-registration nursing education. Online. Available: http://www.nmc-uk.org/aFrameDisplay.aspx?DocumentID=328 10 Sept 2006

Nursing and Midwifery Council 2008 The NMC code of professional conduct: standards of conduct, performance and ethics for nurses and midwives. Online. Available: http://www.nmc-uk.org/aFrameDisplay.aspx?DocumentID=3954 6 June 2008

Nursing and Midwifery Council 2005a Standards of proficiency for pre-registration nursing education. NMC, London

Nursing and Midwifery Council 2005b Statistical analysis of the register 1 April 2004–31 March 2005. Online. Available: http://www.nmc-uk.org 5 May 2005

Nursing and Midwifery Council 2006 Standards to support learning and assessment in practice. NMC, London

Nursing and Midwifery Council 2007 A–Z advice sheets: confidentiality. Online. Available: http://www.nmc-uk.org/aFrameDisplay.aspx?DocumentID=1560 13 Aug 2007

Peach L 1999 Fitness for practice. UK Central Council for Nursing, Midwifery and Health Visiting, London

Royal College of Nursing 2005 Guidance for mentors of student nurses and midwives. Royal College of Nursing, London

Thompson I E, Melia K M, Boyd K M 2000 Nursing ethics. Churchill Livingstone, Edinburgh

Viens C, Lavoie-Tremblay M, Leclerc M M, Brabant L H 2005 New approaches to organizing care and work. Health Care Manager 24(2): 150–158

Weston M 2001 Coaching generations in the workplace. Nursing Administration Quarterly 25(2):11–21

Wright C, Rowe N 2005 Protecting professional identities: service user involvement and occupational therapy. British Journal of Occupational Therapy 68(1):45–47

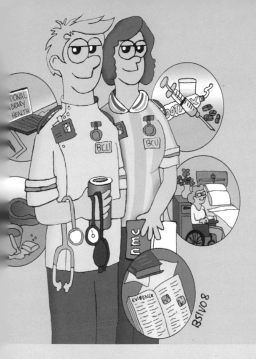

Chapter 2

Great expectations

That was a memorable day to me, for it made great changes in me.
Pause you who read this, and think for a moment ... on one
memorable day ...

Charles Dickens (1812–1870), *Great Expectations*

Introduction

This chapter gives you insights into what you can expect when you
undertake clinical placements and what others will expect of you.
We consider these issues from multiple perspectives as we describe
the expectations of the key stakeholders – the views of patients,
clinicians and professional organizations are explored in detail. We
also discuss your rights and responsibilities as a student and specifically your right to ask questions and to question practice.

2.1 Patients' expectations

What do patients expect from their nurse? This should be a very easy question to answer. Ask your friends, family and fellow students this question and you are bound to get a wide range of responses. What nursing attributes do you think are most important to patients?

We know from a variety of studies carried out over the past 15 years that the skills of caring, empathy, listening, 'being with', comforting, intuiting, assessing, planning and communication are the qualities that patients value most highly (McCormack et al 1999). However, the saying 'The patient doesn't care how much you know, the patient wants to know how much you care' is not always true. Certainly patients want to be able to depend on you to take care of them with kindness and empathy, but with the increasingly complex world of health care, patients want to be sure that you know what you are doing and why you are doing it.

So what does this mean for students? If patients expect to be cared for by nurses with expertise and experience, how do students gain opportunities to learn and practise? You'll be relieved to know that, on the whole, patients are very tolerant of students. If you fumble the first few times when taking a temperature or blood pressure, patients will usually understand. When you are slow at doing a dressing or removing an intravenous line, they will make allowances because you are still learning. Patients will not expect you to be able to answer all their questions, but they will expect you to find someone who can.

There are some things that patients do not make allowances for, irrespective of the nurse's experience or level. Patients expect a student nurse to be as respectful of their privacy as any other nurse. They expect you to be honest about what you know and don't know, and can and can't do. They expect you to be courteous and to treat them with dignity at all times. Even though you are a learner, patients still expect you to carry out procedures safely and accurately, and to acknowledge your limitations.

Patients often comment that they appreciate being cared for by students, because students take the time to stop and talk. In busy hospital units this is often undervalued. Many patients also like to feel that they have been involved in the clinical education of student nurses and will happily explain their history, diagnosis, treatment regimen and medications. Listen carefully: without doubt, you will learn a great deal from your patients – they are the experts about their lives and health conditions. Listen to them, learn from them, and appreciate their stories, for they contain a wealth of information.

Coaching tips

- Make sure you are prepared before you encounter a patient. It is very disconcerting for a patient when a student has no idea of what they are doing, or why. If you are giving a subcutaneous injection, for example, review the procedure; discuss the details with your mentor, and ask as many questions as necessary, before you approach your patient.
- Admit when you are out of your depth. If an infusion pump is sounding an alarm and you don't know how to deal with it, don't stand there for 5 minutes hoping you'll get a moment of inspiration. Find someone who can assist you (then watch and learn).
- If you are taking a blood pressure or any other observation, and you are really not sure whether your result is correct, be honest and ask someone to check it for you.
- Remember that, although technical competence is essential, nursing should not be reduced to a series of tasks lacking the therapeutic qualities that are so important to patients.

2.2 Clinicians' expectations

Over the years we have found that clinicians have the following expectations of nursing students undertaking a clinical placement. Take some time to think about each of these points. Students should:

- understand the nursing context and work they are involved in
- know when to ask for help
- know where to go for help
- recognize their own limitations and deficits
- demonstrate commitment to the nursing team
- ask questions and question practice
- be critically thinking problem-solvers
- be enthusiastic, motivated and positive
- work at becoming proficient in essential nursing skills
- utilize time-management skills
- take advantage of learning opportunities
- be open to the suggestions and guidance offered
- be aware of, and practise within, their scope of practice
- have good interpersonal skills
- practise according to occupational health and safety guidelines
- understand the importance of accurate documentation and other legal and ethical issues

- come to the clinical placement adequately prepared (with clear and realistic clinical learning objectives).

Do these expectations seem realistic to you or a pretty tall order? How do you measure up? It is always interesting, and sometimes surprising, to see a situation from another person's perspective. When the situation is as important as your clinical placement, it is vital that you consider it from many perspectives. We have spent time with many students who were really not aware of what clinicians expected of them, and were puzzled and often hurt by the feedback they received. It is important to build rapport with your mentor at an early stage and to ask if he or she will point out when you are going wrong so that you can rectify it. Take this as constructive feedback and learn from it.

2.3 Professional expectations

In the UK, the professional expectations of nurses are spelt out very clearly. Nurses are required to provide high-quality care through safe and effective clinical practice. Protecting the public through professional standards is an imperative for the Nursing and Midwifery Council (NMC) (Peate 2006). The NMC code of professional conduct (NMC 2008) is reviewed regularly to ensure that the standards are reflective of contemporary practice. The standards state that registered nurses, midwives and specialist community public health nurses are personally accountable for their practice. A shared set of values for all UK healthcare regulatory bodies states that, in caring for patients and clients, you should (NMC 2008):

The people in your care must be able to trust you with their health and wellbeing. To justify that trust, you are required to:

Make the care of people your first concern, treating them as individuals and respecting their dignity:

- Respect people's confidentiality
- Collaborate with those in your care
- Ensure you gain consent
- Maintain clear professional boundaries.

Work with others to protect and promote the health and wellbeing of those in your care, their families and carers, and the wider community:

- Share information with your colleagues
- Work effectively as part of a team

- Delegate effectively
- Manage risk.

Provide a high standard of practice and care at all times:

- Use the best available evidence
- Keep your skills and knowledge up to date
- Keep clear and accurate records.

Be open and honest, act with integrity and upload the reputation of your profession:

- Act with integrity
- Deal with problems
- Be impartial
- Uphold the reputation of your profession.

(Taken from NMC Standards of conduct, performance and ethics for nurses and midwives, 2008)

This code communicates to the general public, particularly the patient, the standards, conduct, performance and ethics expected of nurses. These are the professional expectations that form the framework against which your practice will be assessed. You will be required to demonstrate that you have met these standards as an indication that you are fit to provide safe, proficient care in a variety of settings. Your ability to meet these standards determines your eligibility for registration.

2.4 Don't apologize for being a student

There are three aspects that we'd like to focus on in this section: being proud to be a nurse (or a nursing student), behaving in a way that demonstrates that pride, and apologizing for being a student. So many times students respond to questions from clients, doctors and nursing staff with a self-deprecating answer. When asked, 'What do you do?', 'Who are you?' or 'What is your position?', students often answer, 'Oh, I'm *just a student*'. Likewise, we've heard students (and registered nurses) say to patients, 'Hello. I'm Jill and I'll be looking after you today'. Nurses do so much more than simply *look after* clients. The nursing profession is a proud profession (and rightly so), but for too long nurses have failed to demonstrate real pride in who they are and what they do.

You may not be a registered nurse (yet), or an employee of the institution, but you do have a right to be there, to engage in client-centred activities, to ask questions and to learn. You do not need to apologize for being a student or for being in the clinical learning environment. In fact, you should be proud of your role and the valuable contribution that you make.

Coaching tips

- Practise sharing with others who you are and what you do, in a succinct and professional manner. Put a positive spin on your statements and express pride in your role as a student nurse; for example, 'I am Jill Jones. I'm a third-year nursing student from the university. I'll be working with Bill Smith today and we'll be responsible for your care'.
- Don't apologize when you cannot undertake a clinical skill or activity that you have not previously learnt. Simply explain that you have not been taught that particular skill, but that you would value the opportunity to watch the registered nurse undertake the procedure.
- Similarly, don't apologize for declining when you are asked to do something that you are not legally permitted to do, for example titrating intravenous fluids without supervision. Explain your programme requirements and scope of practice, and politely decline to undertake the procedure.
- Don't apologize for asking questions or for the extra time that mentoring a student takes. Certainly acknowledge and appreciate this, but be mindful that in many respects students are an asset to the clinical staff they work with.
- Lastly, give the people you work with and the clients you are responsible for the respect they deserve, and expect to be treated with respect in return.

2.5 Speak up, speak out

Standing up for what you believe in is one of the most important aspects of personal integrity. Yet speaking up or speaking out is not always easy. Traditionally nursing students were socialized to obedience, respect for authority and loyalty to the team. Their acceptance into, and continued membership of, the healthcare team depended upon their recognition of this subordinate role (Kelly 1996).

Something to think about...

To everything there is a season, and a time to every purpose under heaven: a time to keep silence, and a time to speak.

(Ecclesiastes 3:1)

Nearly a century ago Florence Nightingale described the qualities of a 'good nurse' as 'restraint, discipline and obedience. "She [*the nurse*] should carry out the orders of the doctors in a suitably humble and deferential way. She should obey to the letter the requirements of the matron and the sister" (Davies 1977, p 480). Society expected nurses to be servile, subordinate, humble and self-sacrificing. Within the hierarchy of the healthcare system, nurses became acculturated to do and say what was expected, to conform rather than to question, to accept rather than debate important issues.

Nurses are shaking off this outdated image of nursing, and there are glimpses of a new era on the horizon. But, for some, it is a slow and difficult journey. Little wonder, then, that even today some nursing students find it difficult to speak out when their acceptance into the team may hinge on their conformity to it. There is nothing wrong with wanting to fit in and be accepted – it is a natural social phenomenon (Baumeister & Leary 1995). However, when fitting in becomes more important than doing what is right, it can become an ethical dilemma. The greatest threat to personal integrity is silence in the face of perceived wrong. We sometimes fail to consider the price of silence. To know something is wrong and to say nothing indirectly consents to what has occurred. In doing nothing we become part of the problem. This presents an enormous dilemma for students. By speaking out you may risk ridicule, rejection or social isolation. By not speaking out you may compromise your integrity (or even put somebody's life at risk).

Coaching tips

Many situations may present ethical dilemmas for student nurses. Horizontal violence (or workplace bullying), compromised clinical practice, or breaches of legal and/or ethical standards may call upon you to take a stand and to speak out. How will you respond? What will you say?

The ability to state your opinion clearly and honestly without offending anyone requires great skill. Start by using 'I' statements.

Griffin (2004) provides some excellent examples of 'I' statements for when horizontal violence looms its ugly head:

- 'I don't feel right talking about him/her when I wasn't there and I don't know all the facts.'
- 'I'm not prepared to talk about it as it was shared in confidence.'
- 'I don't think that was what really happened – let's ask the people involved.'

Concerns about patient care standards are just as challenging and often need to be interpreted in consultation with an experienced and objective support person, such as your clinical mentor. Be careful! Sometimes what may seem at first to be poor practice may not be so when interpreted in the light of all the facts. Don't jump in without some guidance and knowledge of all the pertinent issues. You can still use 'I' statements, but be tactful in your approach. 'I don't understand the reason for that decision' is often a wise opening statement that allows for lines of communication to remain open and for explanations to be provided.

There may come a time when you feel you must speak out strongly against a clinical, ethical or professional issue. Make sure you are familiar with and guided by the NMC code of professional conduct (NMC 2008), which provides guidelines for nurses. As a student you may need to call upon your support networks, mentors or educational institution staff for guidance and advice. In some situations they may need to advocate on your behalf.

Speaking up or speaking out is an act of moral courage. It often carries a price tag, but an even greater price tag comes with silence – the loss of self-respect. The benefits of speaking up outweigh the risks, not only from a personal point of view but also for the nursing profession (Kelly 1996; NMC 2007).

When in doubt about whether you should speak out, reflect on the words of Martin Luther King Junior: 'He who passively accepts evil is as much involved in it as he who helps to perpetrate it. He who accepts evil without protesting against it is really cooperating with it.'

2.6 Exercise your rights

In clinical practice experiences, and even in this book, you'll hear a great deal about your responsibilities. Always keep in mind that alongside responsibilities there are also rights. Nurses have focused on their responsibilities for so long that they are often surprised at the prospect of having rights themselves. Rights always seem to belong to other people – human rights, patients' rights, women's rights, consumers' rights – the list goes on. It's time to think about your rights as a nursing student. In this section we'll touch on a few of your rights and provide some strategies to help you to exercise these rights.

Coaching tips

The right to ask questions
As a student, your primary purpose in undertaking a clinical placement is to learn. This won't happen unless you ask questions. Some of the nurses you work with will welcome your questions. These nurses should be congratulated for supporting your learning. Unfortunately, some nurses imply that students ask too many questions.

It's your right to ask questions, but always ask at the right time and in the right place. To develop your problem-solving skills, attempt to work through the question first and develop a tentative answer yourself. For example, you could ask your mentor if your patient's urine output needs to be measured. Alternatively you could check the patient's chart, look for a fluid balance chart, reflect on what may have been said at handover (did you take notes?) and consider the patient's diagnosis (renal failure, congestive cardiac failure, etc.). Doing this allows you to demonstrate initiative and develop an 'informed' question. For example, 'I've measured Mrs Smith's urine output and tested the specific gravity because she has renal failure. Would you like me to document the amount on her fluid balance chart?'.

The right to question practice
This is a right that nursing students don't always exercise. You will learn about 'best practice' and 'evidence-based practice' (and we discuss it in Chapter 3), but at times you will see nursing practice that seems to be based on little more than authority ('The doctor said to do it this way'), tradition ('We've always done it this way') and local policy ('This is the way we do it here'). You may find yourself placed in a confusing and somewhat uncomfortable position with this contradiction between theory and practice.

A student who was undertaking a third-year practice experience, on completing a central line dressing, asked, 'Why is this central line being dressed daily with a gauze dressing? Everything I've read suggests that a transparent dressing that stays on for up to 7 days is the ideal dressing product for central lines'. Now, if you've done any reading about central lines, you'll know that this student was absolutely right! Her comment promoted a lot of dialogue and debate among the registered nurses and doctors. Following a review of the literature, the central line dressing regimen was updated at that hospital. You guessed it – transparent dressings are now used. When questioning practice, remember to be tactful and polite; there may be very sound reasons for the way particular nursing procedures are undertaken.

The right of refusal (without feeling guilty or making excuses)
Often, when students refuse a request from a senior nurse, they feel guilty and uncomfortable, even when they are within their rights – and even when it is their responsibility to refuse. Here is an example in which a student nurse refused, politely and tactfully, but with determination:

Registered nurse: *You can go and administer the oral medications to the patient in room 11. I trust you.*
Student: *Thank you for trusting me to do this on my own, but as a student I'm required to have the administration of all medications counterchecked, witnessed and countersigned by the nurse responsible for the patient's care. I can fail my clinical placement if I don't comply with this policy.*

The right to be supernumerary to the workforce
Since nursing education moved to institutions of higher education, students have undertaken clinical placements in a supernumerary capacity. This means that you are not part of the workforce but are there *in addition* to the employed staff. This is so that your learning is not compromized by the demands and responsibilities of patient care. However, students, particularly when in third year, are occasionally used to fill a gap in staffing. Although we encourage students to take a patient load, it should always be under the supervision of the nurse responsible for the patient's care. If this situation presents itself, politely explain your educational institution's policy.

2.7 You're not the boss of me (oh really?)

As you step into your next ward, excited and ready to begin your clinical placement, the sister in charge will be there, standing at the door, smiling in welcome, eager for you to feel wanted and needed. She or he will spend much time complimenting you on your skills and making wonderful comments about you to the other staff. She or he will most definitely understand when you are late for your shift because of car problems, or not in correct uniform because you 'forgot' to do the washing, or when you seem a little tired or unmotivated – after all, nursing is a difficult and tiring occupation, and special allowances do need to be made for students. Reality check! Nurses are busy people. Their first responsibility is patient welfare. Ward managers are responsible for budgets, equipment, resources, standards of practice, occupational health and safety, off-duty, staffing issues and problems, quality management, infection control – the list goes on. Students are just one of the many important considerations for senior nursing staff. They will expect you to meet the same professional standards as their staff in terms of presentation, punctuality, work ethics, standards of practice, etc.

We've heard students complain when they have been reminded by the sister in charge 'not to be late', to 'wear the correct uniform', or to 'tie their hair up'. Some students believe that because they are not employees the clinical staff have no authority over them. You need to be aware that you are a guest in each clinical venue. The person in charge is responsible for all that occurs in the unit, is committed to maintaining high professional practice standards and has the final say on who does (and does not) undertake a placement experience there.

Coaching tips

There are many different leadership styles. No two nurses are alike. Some are hands on, delving into patient care whenever they get the chance. Others prefer to delegate. Some are social, warm and chatty; others are quiet and distant. However, there are some consistencies that you should be aware of.

- Most nurses who are responsible for a ward don't like surprises and don't like to be told about the deterioration of a patient's condition after it has already happened. They want to know when a difficult situation is developing with a patient, rather than have to face an emergency as they are about to go home. They like to be kept informed. Whether equipment is faulty, a patient's false teeth are missing or the cleaners have gone on strike, the 'buck stops' with them, and he or she needs to be kept informed.

- Most nurse managers don't like to be presented with a problem, complaint or concern without some form of proposed solution. It is important to remember that they try to be fair, but they are accountable to the patients, staff, doctors and the administration. Sometimes they really are the 'meat in the sandwich', as there are so many people they must try to satisfy. Managers need to take a global perspective, so be understanding when your needs are not their first priority.
- Many nurses in charge prefer the direct approach. Nothing is more disconcerting (and likely to cause tension and distrust) than hearing about problems through rumours, innuendo and gossip. The direct approach allows for face-to-face discussion of feelings and issues. Choose the most appropriate time and place to bring up difficult or controversial issues.
- Assertiveness is a good communication skill; however, ensure that your information is correct before you speak (and avoid aggressive outbursts).

2.8 Don't take everything personally

The clinical learning environment is a complex social setting (Hughes 2002) that presents countless challenges to students. Some of these you will find exhilarating, and others will provide you with experiences that will help you to improve your interpersonal skills. Accepting constructive feedback from mentors and clinical staff about your behaviour during challenging situations will add to your growth and development. Avoid taking things personally. Some situations that students find themselves in are not always planned, and it is helpful to consider each situation as a clinical issue or problem, rather than something that is a personal attack or problem for you.

Remember that all situations create learning, and through learning we change and grow, develop new skill sets, knowledge and attitudes, and re-evaluate our belief systems. Identify what it is that you know and what it is that you need to seek help with. Compare each situation with previous learning situations and your observations of experienced staff.

Consider this example by a student who demonstrated less than appropriate professional behaviour, following a directive from her clinical mentor.

Evelyn wanted to go to theatre, but she was told by her clinical mentor that she was to remain on the medical ward because the perioperative unit already had a group of students. During the lunch break, Evelyn found out that another student in her group had been to theatre that morning with her patient. She went to her clinical mentor complaining that she had stopped her from achieving one of her goals and that she was favouring other students. Discussions about the situation between Evelyn and her clinical mentor became strained when Evelyn could not understand why she couldn't go to the unit when her fellow student had done so. Evelyn saw the issue as one that was a personal attack on her and complained to university staff about the way she was treated by her clinical mentor.

On examination of the issues surrounding the complaint, the university staff identified that eight students from another university were allocated to the perioperative environment. Students from the ward locations were permitted to visit the perioperative environment only if they accompanied the patients they were caring for. As Evelyn was on a medical ward, none of her patients was scheduled for theatre.

The very nature of the clinical environment is dynamic, and each student's learning experience will be different. It is not beneficial to compare your experiences and opportunities with those of other students, as no two experiences will ever be the same. In the above situation, Evelyn's placement did not give her the opportunity to go to the perioperative unit and it was a professional decision taken by her mentor, not a personal attack.

Coaching tips

- Identify challenging or difficult situations and work through them using conflict resolution skills (see Section 3.4).
- Seek out strategies to help you deal with difficult people or with difficult situations (counselling courses can be beneficial to help with the development of strategies).
- Be aware of your own behaviours, how you react to situations and how you work through issues.
- Seek assistance from mentors and other relevant staff, as necessary, to work through situations in the clinical learning environment.

2.9 Compliance and compromise

This tale revisits the importance of belonging, but delves into the 'dark side' of this phenomenon for nursing students. There is a broad range of psychological literature that describes the importance of belonging, as well as the negative emotional, psychological, physical and behavioural consequences of having this need thwarted. The absence of meaningful interpersonal work relationships can lead to unquestioning agreement with other people's decisions, acquiescence, compliance or going along with negative behaviours sanctioned by group members in order to belong (Clark 1992; Hemmings 1993).

What does this mean for nursing students? Some studies claim that, for many students, the need to belong and to be accepted into the team is more important than the quality of care they provide and the level of competency they aspire to (Bradby 1990; Champion et al 1998; Tradewell 1996). *Reread that sentence a couple of times and ask yourself if it could apply to you.* Nursing students have described how they sometimes go along with clinical practices that they know to be wrong so as not to 'rock the boat'. They share how it is easier just to accept that 'this is the way it is done here' than to be labelled a 'troublemaker' (Levett-Jones 2007). Compare these notions with what you've learnt about questioning practices that are not evidence based.

Coaching tips

We would like to give you a tried and tested recipe for overcoming the need to conform in order to belong, but really there is no simple solution. The best advice that we can offer is that you reflect on this section thoughtfully. At some stage you may be in a situation where you'll feel pressured to compromise your practice: think carefully about the consequences, for you and for your patient.

> **Something to think about...**
>
> *Will you be a change agent or a conformist?*
> *Will you stand up for what you know to be right,*
> *or will you bow to peer pressure?*

2.10 Being naive

Student nurses may not have cornered the market on naivety, but they often take what people say at face value. Some clinical staff may find naivety refreshing in a person just beginning their career. It may motivate them to take the newcomer 'under their wing' and tell them 'how things work around here'. Students tend not to probe deeply to determine the veracity of what they're told, perhaps because they want to see the best in people, or because they don't feel it is their place to do so. Understandably, it is difficult to see the big picture when you are on a placement for only a short period of time.

Coaching tips

- Don't be 'too grateful' when the person who offers to 'show you the ropes' shares titbits of information that undermine other staff on the nursing team.
- Don't feel that you have to take sides or show allegiance to the person who 'takes you under their wing'. In fact, you should avoid this at all costs, maintain a neutral stance and don't get involved in 'office politics'.
- Without assuming the worst, get into the habit of asking yourself what a person's motives might be.
- Don't rely on the word of just one person – always look at the 'big picture'. Gather as much information as possible.
- Trust your instincts – if you feel uncomfortable about what you're being told, it may be for good reason.
- Keep in mind that the type of person who undermines, criticizes and gossips about other staff on the ward may treat you the same way the next time your back is turned.

2.11 Practice experiences at distant locations

If you have the opportunity to undertake a practice experience in another health service or country, you are very fortunate. There is nothing like this type of experience to open your eyes to new possibilities. However, preparing for a practice experience at a distance from where you live or study can be very daunting. Just like any other trip, you'll have travel and accommodation details to organize, as well as a host of other practical issues to sort out. On top of this there may be social and cultural differences between you, your co-workers and your clients to consider. Undoubtedly policies and procedures will be different from those you are used to and you won't have the immediate back-up of academic staff. As if negotiating these issues isn't enough, you will need to consider the learning opportunities available and your specific clinical objectives.

Undertaking a practice experience at a distance can produce a lot of anxiety and this can impact on your learning and your ability to make the most of your experience. We outline here some strategies to help you through what can be a challenging time.

Coaching tips

Preparation

- Think about the type of practice experience that would suit you best, that you can afford and that you are passionate about.
- Distant placements can be expensive – look at all types of travel and accommodation options. Sharing expenses with fellow students may be possible. Investigate whether your educational institution or nursing organizations provide any financial support.
- Don't leave it to the last minute to get organized. This type of experience can take months to organize.
- Preparation requires research. Search on the intranet and internet, and ask at travel agencies. Most importantly, talk to lecturers and students who have been to distant placements. Ask lots of questions to get a realistic picture of what to expect.
- You'll need to know about professional insurance, accommodation options, parking, internet and library facilities, what to wear, who your contact person will be, what area you'll be working in, what they'll expect of you, what you'll be allowed to do.
- Make sure that you have a clear set of learning objectives (see Section 3.12 for more information about clinical objectives), and that you discuss your expectations and learning objectives early in the placement.

When you arrive

- Be positive and enthusiastic. Let the people you work with know that you are pleased to be there, ready to work and motivated to learn.
- Define your student role – in some places you may be expected to just 'tag along', in others to work as part of the team.
- Be open to and welcoming of serendipitous learning opportunities.
- Keep a journal or reflective diary – write down the things you encounter and your reactions to them all. This will help you maintain perspective and will be great to look back on.

- Maintain contact with your mentor. Keep the dialogue open and don't be afraid to ask lots of questions. If you are finding it difficult to meet your learning objectives, discuss this early so that an alternative learning plan can be organized.
- Know when and where to seek help, and don't hesitate to do so.
- Work to resolve conflict (for strategies, see Section 3.4).
- Be prepared for something to go wrong. It is unusual for practice experiences to proceed without a hitch. Laugh; keep your sense of humour. Try to see something of value in each new problem and challenge.

Reflective thinking activities

What is the most important piece of advice that you would give to students about to undertake their first clinical placement?

_____

_____

_____

List your five tips for success when undertaking a clinical placement experience:

1. _____

2. _____

3. _____

4. _____

5. _____

Have you ever been in a clinical situation where you believed patient safety or quality care was compromised? What did you do? In hindsight, would you (could you) have done anything differently?

_____

_____

_____

References

Baumeister R, Leary M 1995 The need to belong: desire for interpersonal attachments as a fundamental human motivation. Psychological Bulletin 117(3):497–529

Bradby B 1990 Status passage into nursing: another view of the process of socialisation into nursing. Journal of Advanced Nursing 15:1220–1225

Champion B, Ambler N, Keating D 1998 Fitting in: becoming an insider: a nursing perspective (unpublished report). Nurses Registration Board of New South Wales, Newcastle

Clark C 1992 Deviant adolescent subcultures: assessment strategies and clinical interventions. Adolescence 27(106):283–293

Davies C 1977 Continuities in the development of hospital nursing in Britain. Journal of Advanced Nursing 2(5):479–493

Griffin M 2004 Teaching cognitive rehearsal as a shield for lateral violence: an intervention for newly licensed nurses. Journal of Continuing Education in Nursing 35(6):257–264

Hemmings L 1993 From student to nurse. Paper presented to the Research in Nursing: Turning Points Conference. Conference Proceedings of the National Conference, Glenelg

Hughes C 2002 Issues in supervisory facilitation. Studies in Continuing Education 24(1):57–71

Kelly B 1996 Speaking up: a moral obligation. Nursing Forum 31(2):31–34

Levett-Jones T 2007 Belongingness: a pivotal precursor to optimising the learning of nursing students in the clinical environment. Unpublished PhD thesis, University of Newcastle, Newcastle

McCormack B, Manley K, Kitson A et al 1999 Towards practice development: vision or reality? Journal of Nursing Management 7:255–264

Nursing and Midwifery Council 2008 The NMC code of professional conduct: standards for conduct, performance and ethics for nurses and midwives. Online. Available: http://www.nmc-uk.org/aFrameDisplay.aspx?Document ID=3954 6 June 2008

Nursing and Midwifery Council 2007 Whistle-blowing. Online. Available: http://www.nmc-uk.org/aFrameDisplay.aspx?DocumentID=1595 13 Aug 2007

Peate I 2006 Becoming a nurse in the 21st century. John Wiley, Chichester

Tradewell G 1996 Rites of passage: adaptation of nursing graduates to a hospital setting. Journal of Nursing Staff Development 12(4):183–189

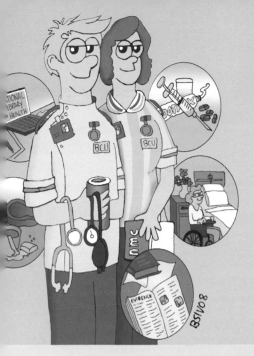

Chapter 3

How you act

Actions speak louder than words.

Proverb

Introduction

This chapter focuses on your behaviour when undertaking clinical placements. We have avoided being too prescriptive by instead profiling some clinical scenarios to help you consider the potential consequences of your actions, good or bad. We've also explored some of the more challenging situations that students may have to deal with, such as sexual harassment, horizontal violence or conflict with peers. Our aim is to fortify you so that if you encounter any of these negative and distressing situations you will have an armoury of strategies to help you deal with them. Our motto is 'forewarned is forearmed'.

3.1 Cultural competence

An increase in cultural diversity in the UK has created the need for nurses to provide culturally competent health care (Watson et al 2002). This presents challenges for nurses as they manage complex differences in attitudes, religion, world views, theories, socio-economic background and language (Kikuchi 2005; Schim et al 2005). The nurse-theorist Madeleine Leininger (1991, p 36) defined culture as people's 'learned and transmitted values, beliefs and practices'. Cultural competence is described as 'the demonstration of knowledge, attitudes, and behaviours based on diverse, relevant, cultural experiences' (Schim et al 2005, p 355). Knowledge of other peoples' culture, beliefs and backgrounds is, therefore, vitally important. To be culturally sensitive you need to recognize the attitudes, values, beliefs and practices within your own culture so that you can have an insight into your effect on others.

When you undertake placements, culturally competent health care means making decisions based on principles such as justice and accountability. It centres on the experiences of the patient and is nested with an acceptance of human diversity (Kikuchi 2005; Schim et al 2005). Cultural competence depends on the capacity of the nurse to improve health by integrating culture into the clinical context.

Nursing students themselves represent a culturally diverse group. In different universities, student populations reflect the social demographics. As a population, nursing students at any one UK university can be culturally very diverse. This provides you with the opportunity to gain knowledge and understanding of others, and to integrate this into your nursing care. Despite many people living hybrid lives influenced by different cultures, there is still a lot to learn from one another. Consider this story.

Mrs Asare had recently arrived from an African country and while staying with her daughter had been diagnosed with lung cancer. She had been admitted to hospital for palliative care. Within a few days the cancerous lesions had grown. She began to experience difficulty in breathing and underwent a procedure to remove fluid from her lung. She found this pleurocentesis (fluid tap procedure) very painful. Her doctor explained that the cancer was extremely fast growing, and she was offered radiotherapy and chemotherapy. She was advised that these approaches would give her a little more time, but would not save her life.

Mrs Asare was very fearful of the equipment and technology that was being used to support her health care and believed in care that did not involve modern-day interventions such as chemotherapy and radiother-apy. She expressed this view to her family, stating that she did not want to progress with further treatment. With her family's blessing, she declined the treatment that may have afforded her a longer life, so that she could die according to her beliefs.

What are your thoughts about Mrs Asare's decision and her need to be true to her beliefs?

Coaching tips

- Make cultural competence an everyday component of your practice. Incorporate cultural diversity (knowledge about the diversity in your healthcare area), awareness (knowledge of culture) and sensitivity (attitudes towards others) into your practice.
- Develop culturally competent behaviours by becoming involved with people from different cultures. Learn from others as you care for them.
- Examine policies and implement practices to promote competent care for persons from diverse backgrounds.
- Promote cultural awareness and team building through open and respectful dialogue.
- Tailor your care to meet patients' social, cultural, religious and linguistic needs.
- Use interpreters for care requirements when language barriers are problematic (but consider the sensitivity of the information that is being imparted by a third person).
- Respect personal space and conversational distance by using the appropriate tone of voice.
- Be attuned to non-verbal communication (body language), silence and touch.
- Use communication skills that reflect your sensitivity and willingness to listen to others.
- Accept and value difference and diversity in human behaviour, social structure and culture.

3.2 The value of a smile

History proves the value of a smile. Studies indicate smiles are the oldest form of expressing the desire and willingness to cooperate. Smiles are potent facial expressions that can be detected from as far away as the far end of a football field, making them the most visible facial expressions from a distance.

The first thing that people usually notice when they meet someone for the first time is that person's smile. In fact, the majority of adults consider a person's smile to be very important at an initial meeting. Three out of four people think a smile is important for succeeding in the workplace.

Consider this scenario.

Not so long ago a mentor was completing a student's clinical appraisal. The appraisal was very good and the student was considered proficient, organized and knowledgable. He was punctual, well presented, articulate, asked appropriate questions and worked hard. However, the student's mentor commented, and the other staff agreed, that she did not get the impression that the student had enjoyed the practice experience. He rarely smiled and a few patients had remarked that he did not seem enthusiastic about being a nurse. When this feedback was shared with him, he was taken by complete surprise. He felt that this experience had been the best he'd had so far and he was unaware that he had been perceived in this way. He admitted he was very serious about being a good nurse, but did not realize that his seriousness would be interpreted by others as a lack of enthusiasm and enjoyment.

Coaching tips

When we are in a new environment we often wait until someone smiles at us before we offer a smile. Don't wait – a smile encourages others to communicate with us. It can reassure and show empathy to an anxious relative, comfort a distressed child, show support and encouragement to an apprehensive or weary colleague, and welcome a newcomer.

You might be enjoying your practice experience, but fail to show it. Your face should express what you feel when you wish to connect with others. We are not encouraging you to smile inappropriately or without spontaneity. Just be mindful of how important smiling is, how it can break down barriers and how others will interpret your smile as a sign of enthusiasm.

3.3 Teamwork

Introducing the concept of 'teamwork' is difficult without resorting to platitudes and rhetoric. No doubt as a student nurse you have heard a lot about teams and the importance of teamwork. You have probably worked hard to make sure that you fit into the team. Before long you will graduate and be called upon to be a team leader. But what does teamwork really mean and what is the secret to successful teams?

Life lessons are often found in nature. The story of geese (author unknown) is a tale that will provide enlightenment to this sometimes nebulous concept that we call teamwork.

Tale 1

As each goose flaps its wings it creates 'uplift' for the birds that follow. By flying in a 'V' formation, the whole flock achieves a greater flying range than if each bird flew alone.

Coaching tips

There is a lot that we can achieve on our own, and even more can be achieved with the help of colleagues, but the power of what can be achieved by a team is even greater. People who share a common direction achieve great things because they are travelling on the trust of one another. The real world of the nurse is challenging and sometimes difficult. Effective teamwork is essential to nursing because it is the support mechanism that 'lifts and carries' us when we struggle. Alone the problems seem insurmountable; together anything is achievable.

Tale 2

When a goose falls out of formation, it suddenly feels the drag and resistance of flying alone. It quickly moves back into formation to take advantage of the lifting power of the bird immediately in front.

Coaching tips

If we had as much sense as geese, we'd be willing to stay in formation with those who are headed in our direction, be willing to accept their help and advice, and willingly give our support to others. It is difficult being a 'one man show' and there is strength in numbers. Giving help to and receiving help from fellow students and nursing colleagues is what makes a team and makes the impossible seem possible.

Tale 3

When the lead goose tires, it rotates back into formation and another goose flies to the point position.

Coaching tips

Don't be afraid to take the lead and to encourage others. Your leadership may be specific to patient care or provide motivation and a positive direction for the group.

Tale 4

The geese flying in formation honk to encourage those up front to keep up their speed.

Coaching tips

Let others know that they are doing a good job or that you appreciate their feedback. Be positive and encouraging.

Tale 5

When a goose gets sick, wounded or shot down, two geese drop out of formation and follow it down to help protect and care for it. They stay with it until it dies or is able to fly again. Then, they launch out with another formation or catch up with the flock.

Coaching tips

The art of caring is a wondrous human trait. Reach out to others, and show empathy and support to colleagues and peers.

3.4 Managing conflict

Conflict is inevitable and occurs in every workplace and in any relationship. Conflict is difficult and distressing, but it does provide the opportunity for stimulating discussion and for developing your interpersonal skills. Sometimes conflict arises because of a misuse of power, authoritarian tactics or condescension; sometimes it is the result of a misunderstanding or miscommunication; at other times it is simply a personality clash.

Coaching tips

- Ask yourself whether you have done anything to contribute to the conflict. Try to be objective and to look at the problem from all sides.
- Keep things in perspective. This will usually require you to spend some time alone to put your thoughts in order. If the issue is not worth losing sleep over, let it go.
- Confer with the other person in a neutral and private setting (not in the nurses' station).
- Share your thoughts and feelings. Explain the problem from your perspective: 'I feel . . .', or 'It seems to me . . .'.
- Check your understanding. Listen to the other person's perspective. Try to understand the reasons behind the conflict.
- Look for common ground and be willing to attempt a compromise. Pursue a good outcome for all involved. If the other person sees that you are willing to make some changes to achieve reconciliation, they will often meet you half way.
- Try not to become defensive or use personal attacks.
- Consider your tone of voice when discussing your concerns with the person/people involved. You don't want to appear argumentative. Neither do you want to appear timid or nervous.
- Use direct confrontation as a last resort.
- Talk to other students about similar experiences and how they handled them.
- Decide upon a course of action. If a satisfactory compromise cannot be reached, you'll need to make a difficult choice. If you decide to yield to another person's decision, do so without self-pity and resentment. If you decide to stand up for your rights, be aware of relevant policies, the appropriate steps to take, and who to speak to (for example, mentor, tutor or counsellor).

Other considerations

Sometimes other factors affect how you view the situation. Consider whether you are:

- Fatigued – have you been taking care of yourself properly? Could your tiredness be making you unreasonable?
- Stressed – is there something happening in your personal life that is overshadowing your ability to see the situation clearly?

3.5 Dealing with horizontal violence (workplace bullying)

Although many nurses may not be familiar with the term horizontal violence, most have experienced it (and participated in it) at some time during their career (Hutchinson et al 2006). The concept of horizontal violence or workplace bullying has been discussed in the nursing literature for almost two decades. It is defined as nurses covertly or overtly directing their dissatisfaction towards one another and to those less powerful than themselves (Griffin 2004). It has been suggested that, because nurses are dominated (and, by implication, oppressed) by a patriarchal system headed by doctors, administrators and sisters in charge, nurses lower down the hierarchy of power resort to aggression among themselves (Farrell 1997). There are many obvious manifestations of horizontal violence, and others that are quite subtle.

The ten most frequent forms of horizontal violence in nursing (adapted from Duffy 1995; Farrell 1997) are the following:

- non-verbal innuendo (raising of eyebrows, pulling faces)
- verbal affront (snide remarks, abrupt responses)
- undermining activities (turning away, not being available, exclusion)
- withholding information (about practice or patients)
- sabotage (deliberately setting up a negative situation)
- infighting (bickering with peers)
- scapegoating (attributing all that goes wrong to one individual)
- backstabbing (complaining to others about an individual instead of speaking directly to that individual)
- failure to respect privacy
- broken confidences.

Horizontal violence is one of the most personally troubling experiences for nurses. Internationally it is claimed that one in three nurses leave their position because of workplace bullying (Griffin 2004). Students undertaking a practice experience have been identified as a group that is especially vulnerable to horizontal violence. One reason for this vulnerability is their inexperience, which makes their work subject to scrutiny and criticism. Horizontal violence can cause students significant stress, and prevent them from asking questions and feeling that they fit in. Sometimes registered nurses excuse their behaviour by saying, 'This is how people treated me when I was a student'.

Coaching tips

Understanding the origins and extent of horizontal violence in nursing will help you realize that you are not to blame and that you should not take it personally. It is also important that you learn how to break the cycle of horizontal violence by confronting the situation rather than trying to ignore it. Confrontation is difficult, but often results in resolution of the bullying behaviour.

How to confront horizontal violence

Here are some examples of how to confront horizontal violence (adapted from Griffin 2004).

Action: *Non-verbal innuendo (raised eyebrows, face pulling)*
Response: *I sense from your facial expression that there may be something you wish to say to me. It is fine to speak to me directly.*

Action: *Verbal affront (snide remarks or abrupt response)*
Response: *I learn best from people who can give me clear and complete directions and feedback. Could I ask you to be more open with me?*

Action: *Backstabbing*
Response: *I don't feel comfortable talking behind his/her back. (Then walk away.)*

Action: *Broken confidences*
Response: *I thought that was shared in confidence.*

Appropriate behaviours

Here are some appropriate behaviours for those who consider themselves to be professional (adapted from Chaska 2000):

- respect the privacy of others
- be willing to help when asked
- keep confidences
- work cooperatively despite feelings of dislike
- don't undermine or criticize colleagues
- address colleagues by name, and ask for help and advice when needed
- look colleagues in the eye when having a conversation
- don't be overly inquisitive about other people's lives
- don't engage in conversation about a colleague with another colleague
- stand up for a colleague in a conversation if he or she is not present
- don't exclude people from conversations or social activities
- don't criticize publicly

3.6 Dealing with sexual harassment

Some authorities contend that the nursing profession has the highest rate of sexual harassment (Madison & Minichicello 2001). Sexual harassment is perpetuated by both staff and patients, and comes in many guises. Many people tolerate it, some hardly notice it, and some find it amusing in small doses and even laugh about it.

Stereotypical images of nurses have played a contributing part in sexual harassment. Media images of nurses are improving, but in the past nurses were often stereotyped as being flirtatious and sometimes sexually promiscuous. Male nurses have been stereotyped too. They are sometimes victimized for doing what for years was considered to be 'women's work'.

What one person interprets as sexual harassment can be considered by another as a 'bit of harmless fun'. Harassment can run the gamut from offensive jokes or sexual comments to inappropriate touching. Sexual assaults are rare but do occur. The overwhelming majority of sexual harassment cases are between male patients and female nurses (Hamlin & Hoffman 2002). Such harassment creates tension for nurses, who must walk a fine line between meeting their professional responsibilities to patients and protecting themselves.

What is sexual harassment?

Sexual harassment is characterized by conduct of a sexual nature that is unwanted and unwelcome to the receiver. Conduct is considered unwelcome when it is neither invited nor solicited, and the behaviour is deemed offensive and undesirable. Sexual harassment in the workplace is an unlawful exercise of power where the harasser uses his or her authority or power to belittle, intimidate or humiliate (based on Hamlin & Hoffman 2002). Harassing behaviours may include the following (Gardner & Johnson 2001):

- verbal sexual advances determined by the recipient as unwelcome
- sexually oriented comments about someone's body, appearance and/or lifestyle
- offensive behaviour, such as leering, ridicule or innuendo
- display of offensive visual materials
- deliberate unwanted physical contact.

Coaching tips

As a nurse you should be vigilant against sexual harassment. If someone speaks or acts inappropriately towards you, this is what you can do:

- Recognize the behaviour.
- Don't blame yourself.
- Keep a diary of what has happened.
- Tell the person involved that you are uncomfortable with this behaviour and that it offends or scares you. Some people do not realize the effect of their behaviour and are genuinely horrified when they are told that their actions are perceived to be harassing when they thought they were being friendly or amusing. Offenders need to understand that is it not what they intended that matters, but how it is perceived.
- Take yourself out of the situation. If a person seems to be targeting you inappropriately, ensure that you are never alone with them.

- Give no encouragement. If someone is harassing you, don't respond to them. Do not engage in friendly banter.
- Confide in a colleague if you think someone is harassing you, even if it is only minor pestering.
- Know the policies and procedures of the educational and health-care institutions about harassment.
- If the situation escalates, report the offender to your mentor or sister in charge, who can take appropriate action.
- If a patient speaks to you or touches you inappropriately, challenge the person immediately in a firm, clear, loud voice for other people to hear. If the harassment continues, you can ask to have another nurse stand by in the patient's room, or refuse to care for the patient. Regardless of what you do, you should report the behaviour to a superior.

Remember that sexual harassment is against the law. All educational and healthcare institutions have policies to protect against sexual harassment. Do not tolerate it (or perpetuate it) in any form.

3.7 Taking care of yourself

Nursing students are a healing presence to others. It is essential that you care for yourself to enable you to continue to care for others and to practise safe nursing (Stark et al 2005). Caring for yourself requires that you proactively adopt healthier lifestyle choices. Practising healthier lifestyle options will maintain and enhance your health and wellness, and put you in the best possible position to cope with the demands of nursing. You are responsible for your own health, and a holistic assessment of your health and well-being will help you to identify your needs and any problems that require a change in lifestyle. Arm yourself with knowledge about health and wellness, select appropriate strategies and commit to making health choices.

Caring for yourself needs to be a priority before you can care for others. The major components of a healthy lifestyle are physical activity, nutrition, interpersonal relations, spiritual growth and stress management (Stark et al 2005). As a role model for others, you should exemplify a healthy lifestyle.

Coaching tips

- Eat well. Get enough rest. Exercise regularly. Be kind to yourself. Take a few minutes each day just to reflect and dream in solitude. Take this time to renew yourself physically, mentally, emotionally and spiritually. Private time is not a luxury – it is a necessity.

- Assess and analyse your own health. Set up a personalized plan that addresses your needs and problems. Seek professional health advice as necessary. Many gyms will assist you with health advice.
- Ensure that you are familiar with the immunization requirements of the NHS. Most universities require you to have evidence of having complied with these requirements before you are authorized to begin your practice experiences.
- Manual handling injuries are one of the most common reasons for nurses' absenteeism. It is vitally important that you learn safe manual handling techniques and practise these at all times.
- You'll learn a lot about infection control during your studies. Remember that infection control protects both your patients and you!
- Remember that you are only human. This is your greatest strength and greatest weakness. Learn to say no to people who put excessive demands upon you. Learn to say yes to activities you really enjoy.
- Develop time management skills to help you juggle study, friends, family and work. Prioritize and don't leave things to the last minute (the extra stress is just not worth it).
- Implement strategies to lessen the effects of lifestyle and work stressors. Try to eliminate as many of these stressors as possible (for example, learn progressive relaxation).
- Set up support networks with colleagues for placements. These can include childcare support networks, travel groups and study groups. You will need to be proactive to work on this.
- Talk about your placements with one another (remember confidentiality and privacy requirements) – this is a great debriefing mechanism as well as an affirming strategy.
- Seek help and support early in your placement if you perceive a problem. It is better to deal with issues early than to allow them to escalate.

3.8 Patient advocacy

Patient advocacy is an essential responsibility for all health professionals – it is no less an obligation for students. To be an advocate means that you should empower and uphold the rights and interests of others. Patient advocacy is defined as an ethical principle of beneficence and is 'defending the rights of the vulnerable patient, or acting on behalf of those unable to assert their own rights' (Thompson et al 2000, p 20). Ways to advocate for and to empower others could include the following:

- informing a patient of her or his rights
- helping a patient to explore options
- helping patients to help themselves
- speaking on behalf of a patient (if and when requested)
- assisting patients to express their views clearly and confidently
- investigating and following up on complaints.

As well as acting as advocate for others, you may require an advocate yourself at times during your nursing career. In some circumstances your mentor may be able to advocate on your behalf, or your tutor or your professional or union representative may be the person who can best represent your interests. Do not hesitate to request this type of support. You should also be aware that there are professional advocates available, and a search of websites (for example, of professional groups and nurses' associations) will identify services available.

Coaching tips

- Identify the essential human rights that a nurse must respect in order to be a patient advocate.
- Identify your responsibilities as a patient advocate.
- Carefully gather relevant information related to the situation and patient before addressing an issue. Try to stand back from the personal and analyse all issues objectively.
- Empower patients to self-advocate rather than taking over (that is, allow patients to ask their own questions of members of the interdisciplinary healthcare team). Perhaps set the scene so that patients are able to ask their questions, or suggest they write their questions down before a consultation.
- Provide patients with information that enables them to make informed decisions.
- Speak up and seek support for your concerns from your mentor or tutor.
- Use the support of tutors to work through issues and principles that you may be concerned about – follow university policies and procedures related to patient advocacy.

3.9 Best practice

Something to think about. . .

The true journey of discovery does not consist of searching for new territories, but in having new eyes.
Marcel Proust (1871–1922), French novelist

Often when we visit students on a practice experience, we ask them questions like: 'What are you doing?', 'Why are you doing it?', 'Why are you doing it that way?' or 'Is there a better way?' We're always thrilled if they can provide evidence-based justification for their decisions. So often, nursing care is based upon little more than tradition or authority. Let us explain.

As a nursing student you will learn how to practise nursing, and some (hopefully most) of what you learn will be research based. Millenson (1997) estimates, however, that 85% of healthcare practices have not been validated scientifically. Nursing practice relies on a collage of information sources that vary in dependability and validity, and some sources of evidence and knowledge are more important than others (Dawes et al 2005). Let us consider some of these sources.

Sources of evidence and knowledge

Tradition
In the nursing profession certain beliefs are accepted as facts and certain practices are accepted as effective, based purely on custom and tradition. These traditions and customs may be so entrenched that their use and usefulness is not questioned or rigorously evaluated. It is worrying when 'unit culture' (the way it is done here) determines the way practice is undertaken, rather than basing clinical judgement on the best available evidence.

Authority
Another common source of knowledge is an authority figure, a person with specialized expertise and/or in a position of authority. Reliance on the advice of authority figures such as sisters, mentors or academics is understandable. However, like tradition, these

authorities as a source of information have limitations. Authority figures are not infallible (especially if their knowledge is based mainly on personal experience), yet their knowledge often goes unchallenged.

Clinical experience

Clinical experience is a familiar and important source of knowledge. The ability to recognize regularities and irregularities, to generalize and to make predictions based on observations is a hallmark of good nursing practice. Nevertheless, personal experience has limitations also. Individual experiences and perspectives are sometimes narrow and biased.

Intuition

Nurses sometimes rely on 'intuition' in their practice. Intuition is a form of knowledge that cannot be explained on the basis of reasoning or prior instruction. Although intuition and 'hunches' undoubtedly play a role in nursing practice, it is inappropriate to depend solely on these feelings as a source of evidence for practice.

Trial and error

Sometimes we tackle problems by successively trying out alternative solutions. Although this approach may in some cases be practical, it is often fallible and inefficient, to say nothing of the ethical implications of trial and error in clinical practice. This method tends to be haphazard, and the solutions are often idiosyncratic.

Assembled information

In making clinical decisions, healthcare professionals may use information that has been assembled for various purposes. For example, local, national and international benchmarking data provide information on the rates of various procedures and/or related complications (such as hospital-acquired infections). Risk management data such as critical incident reports and medication error reports can be used to assess and measure improvements in practice. However, they do not always provide the actual knowledge needed to implement improvement.

Evidence-based research

Nurses are increasingly expected to adopt an evidence-based practice approach, which can be defined as the melding of current and best evidence with individual clinical expertise that is considerate of patient values to bring about a positive outcome for a patient (Joanna Briggs Institute 2007). Evidence from rigorous studies constitutes the best type of evidence for underpinning nurses' decisions, actions and interactions with patients. Nursing care that is based upon high-quality research evidence is more likely to be cost effective and result in positive outcomes.

The need for evidence to support practice has never been greater. The knowledge on which nursing care is based is constantly changing, and some of what you are taught in your nursing programme will rapidly become obsolete. The volume of literature available to nurses is too large to stay continually up to date, and transferring this research evidence into practice is sometimes difficult. For a nursing student, finding the best evidence for practice may seem daunting.

Fortunately a lot of research has already been conducted, systematically reviewed and critically appraised. Organizations such as the Joanna Briggs Institute, the Cochrane Collaboration and Bandolier among others, provide research for practice in an easy-to-understand format called systematic reviews, best practice information and evidence-based care sheets. These documents provide a summary of the best available evidence. Ask your librarian for advice about the best websites for accessing this type of quality research information.

Something to think about...

Every time you undertake nursing care or make a clinical decision, your action is based on something. It may be something that you have heard or read, or what your intuition tells you is the right thing to do. It is your professional responsibility to ask: 'How do I know that this is really the most accurate decision or action?'. Some practices that are based on information other than research are simply not the best way of doing things.

Coaching tips

Consider some of the procedures that you perform during placement. Where did the knowledge on which you base your practice come from? Are you sure that your knowledge and practice are evidence based?

Activity

Select one of the skills that you have learnt and practised on your clinical placement. Access an evidence-based practice website and review your knowledge and practice in light of the best available evidence. Ask yourself the following questions:

- What are you doing?
- Why are you doing it?
- Why are you doing it that way?
- Is there a better way?
- What is the 'best' way?

3.10 Practice principles

The performance of any nursing skill or procedure is informed by guiding practice principles. From these principles, behaviours can be generated for each nursing skill. The integration of knowledge (theories, concepts, rationales, evidence) within each practice principle forms the foundation of the behaviours for the nursing skill. You can use practice principles as a tool to reflect critically upon your nursing. A set of behaviours for each nursing skill (for example, showering, wound care, assessment of vital signs) can be generated using practice principles.

Table 3.1 identifies a core set of principles that applies to any nursing skill undertaken.

Table 3.1   Practice principles (adapted from Andersen 1991)

Guiding practice principle	Examples of behaviours undertaken and informed from practice principles	Knowledge (e.g. theories, concepts, rationales, evidence)
Establishment of a need	• Assessment of health status • Monitoring changes in the patient • Implementing patient treatment orders (e.g. medication is due)	• Normal health status • Anatomy and physiology • Pharmacokinetics • Administration of medication

table continues

Table 3.1 Practice principles (adapted from Andersen 1991)—Cont'd

Guiding practice principle	Examples of behaviours undertaken and informed from practice principles	Knowledge (e.g. theories, concepts, rationales, evidence)
Establishment of a state of readiness for nurse, patient and equipment	• Explanation to the patient • Checking to make sure the patient has time for the procedure (i.e. patient is not scheduled for an X-ray) • Collection of equipment required • The nurse identifies that the necessary support is available for the procedure (e.g. personnel to help with positioning or to check medications)	• Communication • Time management • Understanding hospital processes • Knowledge about resources and equipment necessary for undertaking the procedure
Maintenance of patients' safety and comfort	• Handwashing technique (social and/or surgical washes) • Providing pain relief before the start of a procedure • Positioning the patient before undertaking the procedure	• Asepsis • Microorganisms • Pain • Pharmacology • Body alignment
Prevention of untoward outcomes	• Providing assistance to the patient as necessary • Ending the procedure (removal of rubbish to prevent cross-infection)	• Respect • Cross-infection
Assessment of patient's participation	• Assessing and/or encouraging the patient to participate • Encouraging self-care • Providing patients' education to promote with their participation in health goals	• Motivation • Assessment of health • Self-care • Patient education • Health • Goal-setting • Ethics

table continues

Table 3.1 Practice principles (adapted from Andersen 1991)—Cont'd

Guiding practice principle	Examples of behaviours undertaken and informed from practice principles	Knowledge (e.g. theories, concepts, rationales, evidence)
Evaluation of the activity in terms of effectiveness and appropriateness	• Assessment of patient and monitoring changes during and following the procedure (e.g. side-effects of drugs) • Evaluation of patient (e.g. comfort)	• Assessment • Health status • Normal structure and function • Pharmacology • Comfort • Caring
Accuracy of reporting and recording	• Reporting outcomes (e.g. handover report) • Recording data and procedure undertaken (i.e. nursing notes)	• Reporting • Recording • Legal considerations • Communication

Activity

• Select one nursing procedure with which you are familiar (e.g. temperature measurement, blood pressure measurement, or showering a patient). Beside each guiding principle in Table 3.1, list the behaviours that you would undertake to perform the selected procedure proficiently. Be specific in describing your actions. To facilitate your learning, cross-check your behaviours with a basic or fundamental nursing text that describes nursing skills (Brooker & Waugh 2007).

• Consider the behaviours associated with each principle for your selected nursing skill. Develop a list of learning issues (knowledge, concepts, research, theories, rationales, etc.) for follow-up that will allow you to expand your knowledge associated with the selected skill.

3.11 Clinical governance

Clinical governance is a framework designed to help clinicians improve quality and safeguard standards of care. It is a fundamental principle that encourages openness about strengths and weaknesses, and incorporates the need to be proactive in order to improve through best practice (Duffy & Irvine 2004; Greco et al 2004). Clinical governance requires accountability and responsibility for quality care (Tait 2004). Clinical governance is about having the right people, policies, processes and information to be effective in delivering health care.

Many quality improvement strategies are implemented in the clinical environment. You may be involved in strategies such as risk management, audits and staff development, where clinical governance frameworks are used as a coordinating mechanism for quality.

The guiding principles of clinical governance include (Tait 2004):

- a focus on continuous quality improvement
- application to all facets of health care, across all service areas, models of practice, and inclusive of all healthcare providers through teamwork and sharing
- development of partnerships between all people involved (patients and their families, sisters in charge, clinicians, students)
- involvement of patients and the public
- learning from mistakes
- openness about failure
- emphasis on learning
- development of a just culture where individuals are treated fairly.

During practice experiences you will find evidence of clinical governance principles being implemented and will certainly be involved in different strategies. Each institution will interpret the principles differently and will implement strategies that have meaning and relevance to the patients, the community and staff in that facility. For example, there may be systems and infrastructure implemented to ensure quality of care, a set of guidelines or standards that you will be required to use, and mechanisms for data collection so that analysis and reports about care provision and services can be generated. In some cases these reports are directly linked to funding for the institution.

Some examples of clinical governance include the following (Duffy & Irvine 2004; Tait 2004):

- management of serious complaints
- performance reviews
- clinical audits
- management of incidents and accidents
- critical incident review
- clinical practice improvement programmes (e.g. care pathways, standard setting)
- education, training and staff development programmes
- accreditation and external quality reviews
- benchmarking processes
- policy generation.

Coaching tips

- Understand the principles of clinical governance.
- Discuss with members of the interdisciplinary team their understanding of clinical governance principles, and how the principles contribute to sharing information and care provision with this framework.
- Actively contribute to strategies that support clinical governance frameworks.
- Reflect upon the shared beliefs and values of the interdisciplinary team. Analyse these with regard to the culture of the clinical learning environment.
- Identify the systems and tools that have been implemented to facilitate quality of care. Question others about how these systems have changed and improved practice (for example, an appraisal system, feedback mechanisms, case management reviews, and education sessions).
- Continually re-evaluate your own practice through reference to standards, evidence-based practice, policy and legislation.

3.12 Clinical learning objectives

When on a practice experience your learning will be both opportunistic and structured. In this section we talk about how clinical objectives help to provide structure and direction to your learning experience. In some ways a set of clinical objectives is like a well thought out itinerary: it guides your clinical journey, keeps you focused on the most important areas and can be used to communicate to others (for example, mentors) what you hope to achieve and where your interests lie. Your clinical objectives may be prescribed or you may be required to develop your own. Either way they should be SMART (Fowler 1998):

- specific
- measurable
- achievable
- realistic
- timely.

Learning objectives help you become a safe, effective, proficient and confident registered nurse. Your objectives will become progressively more sophisticated as you proceed through your programme, and each semester they will build upon and consolidate what you have already learnt.

Coaching tips

When developing your clinical learning objectives you should consider the following questions:

- What do you want to learn (objective)?
- Why do you want to learn it (rationale)?
- How are you going to learn it (strategy)?
- How are you going to prove that you have achieved your objective (evidence)?

An example of a clinical objective

Objective: To become proficient and confident in assessing patients' blood pressure and determining whether it falls within normal parameters for the individual.

Rationale: Assessing blood pressure is a vital nursing skill and an important indication of a patient's haemodynamic and cardiovascular status. This is a skill that I do not feel confident with.

Strategy: I will research best practice guidelines regarding blood pressure assessment, practise the skill when I have the opportunity on placement, and ask for feedback from my mentor.

Evidence: When I feel proficient and confident I will ask my mentor to complete the blood pressure skills assessment form to confirm my achievement of this objective.

Developing learning objectives will require you to reflect upon your previous clinical experiences and review your strengths and limitations. Read Sections 4.2 (Reflective practice) and 4.3 (Reality check and seeking feedback) before you begin to develop your objectives. You will also need to be self-directed and insightful in order to develop objectives that are meaningful and relevant to your stage of development. Use the Nursing and Midwifery Council Standard of Proficiency (NMC 2004) as a benchmark to help you analyse what you already know and can do, and where you need to focus, consolidate, develop and improve. In addition, consider the context of your practice experience and your scope of practice (review Section 1.6: Working within your scope of practice). There is no point in having the objective 'develop knowledge and skills in the management of arterial lines' on your first placement, or when working in an aged care facility. Remember also that your clinical objectives should focus on the development of knowledge, skills *and* attitudes.

Finally, it is wise to discuss your objectives with your mentor, who will be able to determine whether they meet the SMART criteria listed above. It is important to know early on in a placement whether or not your objectives are realistic for your level of experience, and whether you will be able to achieve your objectives in a particular unit, with a particular patient mix, and within a specific time frame. Don't be surprised if your objectives need to be amended slightly.

3.13 Student assessment

The clinical learning environment is an important component of formal learning, and assessment of student clinical performance forms an essential part of the teaching–learning process (Santy & Mackintosh 2000; Watson et al 2002). Assessment allows you to gain a sense of achievement, to gauge your progress and to appreciate your ability to practise in the real world.

Various forms of clinical assessment are used in practice. Some assessments are designed to provide you with ongoing feedback, others determine your proficiency (perhaps in performing a nursing skill), and some may provide a measure of your skills or knowledge based on a set of criteria (Fisher & Parolin 2000; Goldsmith et al 2006; Watson et al 2002). NMC proficiency standards (NMC 2004) underlie many assessments related to clinical performance. For example, you may be required to complete an appraisal of your performance (that is, a self-assessment) before your mentor assesses you, based on the proficiency standards. Other examples of clinical assessments may include the following.

- You may be required to undertake patient transfer techniques with your mentor, who will complete a feedback sheet that becomes a critical element for your portfolio submission. A self-assessment of your transfer technique may also be needed for the portfolio.
- You might be asked to attend to a set of nursing care procedures under supervision, which may then be rated according to best practice guidelines.
- Alternatively, you may be expected to collect data that will form the basis of an assessment item, such as the direct observation of wound healing.

For some assessments, your institution may state that you must be assessed by people who are qualified to assess you (for example, your mentor, practice teacher or teacher). In other situations self-assessment of your clinical performance is also a valuable learning tool. Different approaches to self-assessment are used in nursing programmes across the UK.

There are many competing needs in a clinical learning environment and you should focus on the broader picture rather than your personal needs. You should be considerate of staff workloads and other pressures (Edmond 2001). Remember that care requirements for patients are always paramount and your need to be assessed must not compromise the health or welfare of a patient; on some practice experiences there may be situations or issues that make it difficult for you to undertake your required assessments. Examples of these could occur when:

- There are limited opportunities in the clinical learning environment to allow you to undertake the assessment.
- Your mentor is unable to assess you because of the competing demands of others (for example, patient care demands or other students).
- The number of student assessments to be undertaken does not allow all students the opportunity for practice or supervision.
- Some students require more supervision than others, and these students take more of the teacher's time.

- Students are too slow because they have not taken the time to practise the procedures before their practice experience. The teacher therefore deems that the student is not ready to be assessed at the time of request.

Coaching tips

- Discuss assessment requirements with your mentor or practice teacher early in the placement. You may find that making an appointment prior to your practice experience relieves pending anxiety.
- Communicate any difficulties you perceive about meeting the assessment requirements to the appropriate person (this may be to your mentor, practice teacher or tutor) as soon as you identify them.
- As with all nursing care, the principles of safe practice must be integrated into your assessment.
- Know and use the NMC Standards of Proficiency for Pre-registration Nursing Education (NMC 2004) to inform your practice.
- Take advantage of practice opportunities on campus (such as laboratory sessions) to ensure that you are ready for assessment and related care requirements. Self-assess your performance during these sessions using the statements and cues from the NMC proficiency standards.
- Identify competing needs, organizational, clinical, educational or practical.

3.14 Giving and receiving gifts

In this section we focus on giving and receiving gifts. Although society views gift giving as a normal occurrence to show appreciation, giving or receiving gifts in the context of the nurse–patient therapeutic relationship has the potential to invoke emotional discomfort and embarrassment, and to compromise a relationship where trust, rapport and the power balance may be open to exploitation.

Patients often express their gratitude by giving a small gift at the end of their stay as a gesture of thanks. This type of gift is usually given to one nurse but is accepted on behalf of the team. It may take the form of tokens such as flowers, chocolates or fruit, which are left at the nurses' station for sharing. To avoid breaching policies you could decline a personal gift but accept a small token of appreciation on behalf of the team.

Always assess the appropriateness of any gift that is offered to ensure that the giving of these gifts (or favours) could not be interpreted as being in return for preferential treatment (NMC 2007). There are several factors to consider when a gift is offered:

- the timing of the gift in relation to the patient care episode (before, during or after care is provided)
- the intent of the gift and any expectation of different care being provided as a result of the gift
- the potential consequences of accepting or refusing the gift, such as family responses or any emotional discomfort.

Consider the following story.

Linda had been caring for Mrs Fairford, an elderly woman, for several weeks when suddenly her patient gave her a ring that she had owned since she was 18 years old. She stated that she wanted Linda to have it because she didn't think she would still be around the following week when Linda returned to placement. Linda assured Mrs Fairford that she would see her the following week and at first refused the gift. When Mrs Fairford reasserted her desire for Linda to have the ring, Linda finally accepted.

Mrs Fairford passed away during Linda's days off and when her family came to collect her belongings they noticed that their mother's ring was missing. The family demanded that the ring be found. The patient's room was thoroughly searched, but of course the ring was not found. The sister in charge asked to speak to all staff who had cared for Mrs Fairford. It was at this interview that Linda found out that the ring she had been given by Mrs Fairford had been reported missing by the family. Mrs Fairford had not informed her family of her decision to give Linda the ring, nor had Linda told anyone about her gift.

What are your thoughts about this situation? Was it appropriate for Linda to have accepted the gift? Could Linda have breached any policy or standard of conduct? What impact did this gift have on the family and on Linda?

Coaching tips

- Consider carefully whether you should accept a gift offered by a patient.
- If you do accept a token gift, accept it on behalf of the team.
- Seek advice from your mentor or sister in charge about a gift that is offered by a patient or a patient's family member.

When students want to show appreciation

Another perspective to consider is the giving of gifts by nursing students. Students sometimes feel that they would like to show their appreciation to staff who have been involved in their teaching. When giving a gift, be mindful that you do not place a colleague or supervisor in a position where he or she feels pressured or uncomfortable.

Usually, the best way to offer a gift is as a parting gesture. It may be more appropriate if the gift is offered by a group rather than an individual (this of course depends on the number of students allocated to the mentor or unit). Here are some suggestions for ways to show appreciation:

- Verbal thanks can be expressed directly to your mentor and to the sister in charge of the unit.
- A card or certificate expressing your appreciation can be given. Be specific – name the people who went out of their way for you and say what you gained from your experience.
- A gift such as a pot plant, flowers, a basket of fruit or box of chocolates is always appreciated.
- Some of our students have provided morning tea for the staff on the last day of their placement.

Accepting thanks

It is equally important to accept appreciation from the nursing staff for your contribution. I recently overheard a registered nurse thanking a student for her hard work and telling her that her clinical skills were outstanding. The student's response was to downplay and minimize her success: 'It was nothing', she shyly replied. Minimizing words are those that diminish or deprecate the importance of your achievement. While nurses may not have cornered the market in the use of minimizing words, they certainly use them too often.

- Practise responding to compliments and thanks positively, for example, 'Thank you, it was my pleasure'.
- Don't use words such as 'I only …', 'It was nothing' or 'I just …'.
- If you must be modest, try saying, 'Thank you, I'm pleased with my progress. I really did have a lot of support and guidance from the registered nurses I worked with here'.

3.15 Documentation and legal issues

Quality documentation is a requirement of all healthcare professionals. Documentation may make or break the defence of a hospital and staff if legal action is instigated following a critical incident or unexplained death.

Some points to consider

- Documentation is considered to be the most important evidence in a potential legal action and therefore its significance should never be underestimated.
- Legal action may be initiated many years after a critical incident occurs. Memories of witnesses will obviously fade and therefore accurate documentation may be crucial to the outcome of the case.
- Accurate documentation will ensure that your nursing report demonstrates evidence of the care given to your patients, as well as providing a means of communication between healthcare professionals.
- Accurate documentation means more relevant documentation, not more extensive documentation.
- Quality documentation will save you time and may protect you from potential litigation.
- Remember the best answer to litigation is concise, accurate, objective and contemporaneous documentation.

Coaching tips

- Reports should be concise. Avoid verbosity and 'double charting'. Document only aberrations from normal in the integrated patient notes. Avoid useless and unnecessarily long words and sentences. Use care plans and clinical pathways as adjuncts to integrated progress notes, but do not duplicate information.
- Reports should be accurate. You should distinguish between what you observe personally and what is related to you by another person (hearsay); for example, 'The patient stated that she had slipped over', not 'The patient slipped over'. Unless you have actually witnessed the incident, the patient's complaint is hearsay and must be reported as such.
- Reports should be objective. Avoid using the word 'appears'. You should record what you actually see, not what you think you see;

for example, 'The patient appears to be in shock' should instead be documented as 'The patient is pale and sweating, hypotensive, BP 80/40, tachycardic, pulse 140, with peripheral cyanosis', or 'The patient was observed at 2-hourly intervals during the night, and when so observed was sleeping', not 'Patient appears to have slept all night'.

- Documentation should be contemporaneous. It should be written as close as possible to the time when the incident or treatment occurred. Memories fade and often one incident is followed closely by a series of incidents, particularly if a patient's condition deteriorates and a number of treatments are initiated. Trying to put this in sequence at the end of the shift can be confusing and lead to inaccuracies.
- Always sign and print your name, and include your designation.
- Documentation should be specific. Say exactly what you mean; for example, 'Patient experienced a sudden onset of severe breathlessness following ambulation, respiratory rate 40', not 'Patient feeling breathless'.
- Documentation should be legible, with correct spelling and grammar. Nurses often complain about doctors' handwriting, but nurses, too, may be at fault. If a negligence case is taken to court, your nursing notes may be used as evidence. Imagine how you'd feel if your notes could not be interpreted because of poor legibility. Furthermore, reports filled with misspelt words and incorrect grammar creates the same negative impression as illegible handwriting.
- Document all relevant information. Document any change in the patient's condition, what you observed to support this observation, your follow-up actions, and to whom you notified the change. Do not document normal observations that have been charted elsewhere, such as vital signs, postoperative observations, and voiding or drain patency, but do document if there are any aberrations from normal and what your actions were. The use of clinical pathways and care plans has significantly reduced the need for extensive documentation in the integrated progress notes.
- Only accepted abbreviations are to be used. Nurses work in many different institutions during their practice experiences and later employment. A diversity of abbreviations can lead to confusing and misleading interpretations; for example, the abbreviation SB can be taken to mean 'short of breath' or 'seen by'. Make sure

you understand the meaning of any medical and nursing abbreviations used and include only commonly accepted and easy-to-understand abbreviations in your notes.

- An error should be dealt with by drawing a line through the incorrect entry and initialling it. Total obliteration may suggest that you have something to hide. White-out should not be used, for the same reason.

- Never make an entry in a patient's notes before checking all relevant details to ensure you have the correct patient and his or her corresponding chart. Don't rely on room numbers only. Patients are often moved from room to room, and have also been known to 'get into the wrong bed'.

- All omissions should be documented. If you do not carry out an ordered treatment or procedure, always document why it was omitted and whom you notified. If nothing is written, it may be presumed that the procedure was overlooked. For example, if a patient's hypertensive medication was not administered because the patient's blood pressure was too low, this must be documented in the patient's notes and the medication chart. The follow-up action and the person notified should be included. When you are busy with patient care, documentation may seem to be of secondary importance. However, from a coroner's point of view an incomplete chart may suggest incomplete nursing care. This is not always true, but it is an easy inference to make. You may have performed a nursing procedure and you simply forgot to chart it, but if a dispute arises many years later you will have nothing to back up your version of the facts – assuming you can even remember what you did at the time.

- Be aware that the assumption is made that if something is not documented then it has not been done.

- Never make an entry in a patient's notes of behalf of another person.

- Be aware that nurses are practising in an era of consumerism. This has created a more litigious and complaint-oriented society. In order to protect themselves from potential litigation, nurses need higher quality and more relevant documentation. They should always bear in mind that they will be held accountable for the care provided to patients and may be called upon to explain their actions in relation to patient care. Good-quality documentation is part of a nurse's accountability and may be the only assistance that nurses can rely upon if asked to explain their professional actions.

3.16 Visitors during practice experiences

Practice experiences often require a memorandum of understanding or agreement. These agreements between the educational institution and the healthcare facility set out requirements, restrictions and conditions for the practice experience. Students are therefore bound by specific rules, regulations and policies. As a general principle, students are not to receive personal visitors during practice experience. However, if a personal visit is anticipated, you should discuss it in advance with the appropriate person. Facilities have in place policies that guide special circumstances, such as the needs of breast-feeding mothers.

Coaching tips

- Inform your family and friends that it is inappropriate for them to visit you on practice experience unless it is an emergency.
- Instruct family members about how to contact you in an emergency. Document your placement details (facility, shift, ward and contact number) for urgent contact requirements.
- Ensure that your contact details are current on your educational institution database system (especially emergency contact details).
- If you have unwanted visitors while on practice experience, immediately seek assistance from the sister in charge and/or facility security.

3.17 Using the company supplies

Nursing students undertaking practice experiences enter health facilities where resources are calculated and costed for patient care. Those students who help themselves to health facility supplies contribute to costs associated with the health budget.

You should also consider what is provided by the facility for staff and what they themselves contribute. Consider the following story.

Cathy's practice experience was in a small private clinic. On orientation to the facility, the sister in charge showed Cathy the staff tearoom, but requested that she go to the cafeteria in the next building for all her meal breaks. On the second day of the practice experience, Cathy decided that she couldn't be bothered walking to the cafeteria and helped herself to coffee and biscuits in the staff tearoom. The staff said nothing about her using the tearoom and she continued to have her meal breaks in the staff tearoom for the rest of her placement. Cathy was not aware that some of the staff were annoyed about her using their facilities. She did not know that the tearoom supplies were purchased from a staff fund.

Not all facilities provide supplies for staff tearooms. Although a cafeteria may be available for staff use, the staff may contribute to a social club for personal items to support their working environment. These purchases may include the following:

- tea, coffee, biscuits, milk, sugar and juice
- fruit basket supply
- lunch provisions (bread, butter, spreads, etc.)
- soap and shampoo for showers
- subscriptions to newspapers, magazines, journals.

You should not assume that food, drink and supplies left in a common tearoom are available for your use.

Apart from tearoom supplies, there are other resources you should think about before helping yourself. For example, letterhead stationery is expensive and students should not use it as notepaper. Neither should you use preprinted forms (such as medication charts or observation forms) for this purpose.

Similarly, you should ask permission to use the ward photocopier. Think about what it is you are copying, whether you can access the information somewhere else (for instance, from your own computer through internet links, or from a library) and the amount of paper that may be used. Also be mindful of copyright laws. Photocopying is calculated and contributes to the ward or unit budget.

It should not have to be said, but, for those who are unsure, the health facility is not a place to access supplies for your first aid kit. Removal of supplies from a facility without permission constitutes theft. Similarly, newspapers and magazines should be left for patients and visitors to read.

Coaching tips
- Be organized for your practice experience by ensuring that you take essential equipment with you (notebook, pens, safety equipment, etc.).
- Have a notebook (the size of your pocket) to document important notes (remember to adhere to privacy issues).
- Be prepared to contribute to a ward social fund, especially if you are on a ward or unit for an extended period of time.

Reflective thinking activities

What advice would you give the student in the following scenario?

One of your fellow nursing students is undertaking a 6-week practice experience in an intensive care unit. She confides in you that the husband of an unconscious patient she has been caring for is making her feel very uncomfortable. At first he told her what a lovely, caring nurse she was, and then he began to ask her questions about her personal life – where she lived, if she had a boyfriend, and so on. In the beginning she thought he was just being friendly, but lately he has been standing too close to her when she is caring for his wife, and touching her as she walks past him. She mentioned her discomfort to one of the registered nurses she was working with, but he brushed it off, saying that the man 'probably didn't mean any harm'.

_____

_____

_____

What would you do in the following situation?

It is the first day of your second-year practice experience. You are sitting in the tearoom with some of the nursing staff when another student walks in and asks a question about one of the patients she is caring for. The staff answer her question somewhat impatiently, but when she walks out a few of them begin singing, 'Bring in the clowns . . .'. Laughingly they tell you that they are really tired of the silly questions the other student keeps asking.

_____

_____

_____

References

Andersen B M 1991 Mapping the terrain of the discipline. In: Gray G, Pratt R (eds). Towards a discipline of nursing. Churchill Livingstone, Melbourne, p 95–123

Brooker C, Waugh A 2007 Foundations of nursing practice. Elsevier, Edinburgh

Chaska N 2000 The nursing profession: tomorrow and beyond. Sage, Thousand Oaks

Dawes M, Davies P, Gray A et al 2005 A primer for health care professionals. Elsevier, Edinburgh

Duffy E 1995 Horizontal violence: a conundrum for nursing. Collegian 2(2):5–17

Duffy J A, Irvine E A 2004 Clinical governance: a system. Quality in Primary Care 12:141–145

Edmond C B 2001 A new paradigm for practice education. Nurse Education Today 21:251–259

Farrell G 1997 Aggression in clinical settings: nurses' views. Journal of Advanced Nursing 25:501–508

Fisher M, Parolin M 2000 The reliability of measuring clinical performance using a competency based assessment tool: a pilot study. Collegian 7(3): 21–27

Fowler J (ed.) 1998 The handbook of clinical supervision: your questions answered. Quay Books, Salisbury

Gardner S, Johnson P 2001 Sexual harassment in healthcare: strategies for employers. Hospital Topics 79(4):5–11

Goldsmith M, Stewart L, Ferguson L 2006 Peer learning partnership: an innovative strategy to enhance skill acquisition in nursing students. Nurse Education Today 26(2):123–130

Greco M, Powell R, Jolliffe J et al 2004 Evaluation of a clinical governance training programme for non-executive directors of NHS organisations. Quality in Primary Care 12:119–127

Griffin M 2004 Teaching cognitive rehearsal as a shield for lateral violence: an intervention for newly licensed nurses. Journal of Continuing Education in Nursing 35(6):257–264

Hamlin L, Hoffman A 2002 Perioperative nurses and sexual harassment. AORN Journal 76(5):855–860

Hutchinson M, Jackson D, Vickers M, Wilkes L 2006 They stand you in a corner; you are not to speak: nurses tell of abusive indoctrination in work teams dominated by bullies. Contemporary Nurse 21(2):228–238

Joanna Briggs Institute 2007 JBI levels of evidence. Online. Available: http://www.joannabriggs.edu.au/pubs/approach.php?mde+TEXT 29 Sept 2007

Kikuchi J F 2005 Cultural theories of nursing responsive to human needs and values. Journal of Nursing Scholarship 37(4):302–307

Leininger M M 1991 The theory of culture care diversity and universality. In: Leininger M M (ed.). Culture care diversity and universality: a theory of nursing. National League for Nursing, New York, p 5–68

Madison J, Minichicello V 2001 Sexual harassment in healthcare: classification of harassers and rationalizations of sex based harassment behavior. Journal of Nursing Administration 3(11):534–543

Millenson M L 1997 Demanding medical evidence. University of Chicago Press, Chicago

Nursing and Midwifery Council 2004 Standards of proficiency for pre-registration nursing education. Online. Available: http://www.nmc-uk.org/aFrameDisplay.aspx?DocumentID=328 10 Sept 2006

Nursing and Midwifery Council 2007 Gifts and gratuities. Online. Available: http://www.nmc-uk.org/aFrameDisplay.aspx?DocumentID=1572 13 Aug 2007

Santy J, Mackintosh C 2000 Assessment and learning in post-registration nurse education. Nursing Standard 14(18):38–41

Schim S, Doorenbos A, Borse N 2005 Cultural competence among Ontario and Michigan healthcare providers. Journal of Nursing Scholarship 37(4):354–360

Stark M A, Manning-Walsh J, Vliem S 2005 Caring for self while learning to care for others: a challenge for nursing students. Journal of Nursing Education 44(6):266–270

Tait A R 2004 Clinical governance in primary care: a literature review. Issues in Clinical Nursing 13:723–730

Thompson I E, Melia K M, Boyd K M 2000 Nursing ethics. Churchill Livingstone, Edinburgh

Watson R, Stimpson A, Topping A et al 2002 Clinical competence assessment in nursing: a systematic review of the literature. Journal of Advanced Nursing 39(5):421–431

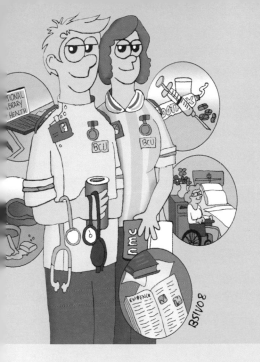

Chapter 4

How you think and feel

If one learns from others but does not think, one will be bewildered.
If, on the other hand, one thinks but does not learn from others,
one will be in peril.

Confucius (551–479 BC), Chinese philosopher

Introduction

This chapter provides an opportunity for you to be introspective, to think consciously and deliberately about your clinical experiences, and to reflect on them in ways that are meaningful, beneficial and action oriented. We show you how to consider your thoughts and feelings carefully, in preparation for, and during and after, your placements. You are also given the opportunity to evaluate your strengths and limitations, to consider feedback provided by others, and to develop strategies for improvement. In this chapter we emphasize that the journey of lifelong learning is the responsibility of every nurse and that learning depends upon your ability to be a reflective practitioner.

4.1 Caring

Nurses enter the nursing profession because they care about people and society. However, nurses don't have the monopoly on caring. Parents care for their children; teachers care about their students; doctors provide clinical care for their patients; chaplains provide pastoral care. So why do professionals view caring differently? Caring is one of those concepts that can be elusive and have different meanings. The literature provides many examples, definitions and theories of caring (Bourgeois 2006; Walsh & Walsh 1999; Watson et al 2002; Williams 1998). For some, caring and nursing may seem to be the same, but others will differentiate caring from nursing.

Nurses understand caring from many perspectives that reflect their experiences, context of practice, and knowledge. One way to understand caring would be to view it as discourses of caring.

Discourses of caring

Discourses are groups of statements that act to constrain and enable what we know (Bourgeois 2006). A finite number of statements contribute to a discourse and these recur time and again, so that we come to see certain statements (often made by very prominent people) as truths. Take, for example, the statement 'Caring is nursing'. This often-repeated statement in the literature is perceived differently by individual nurses.

Three discourses of caring are evident in nursing (Bourgeois 2006) – that is, nurses speak about caring from a position within different discourses, using statements that define and inform others about caring. These discourses are 'caring as being', 'caring as doing' and 'caring as knowing'. Nurses who speak about caring will use statements that belong to these different discourses.

In the discourse 'caring as being', nurses speak about caring as an element that is intrinsic and essential for nurses. Caring for them is part of their nature as human beings, involving them in caring relationships. You may hear some of your peers claim, 'I was born to be a nurse. It is in my family; all my family are nurses', 'Caring is a part of me' or 'All I want is to do is care for others'.

panel continues

Discourses of caring (continued)

The discourse 'caring as doing' is evident when nurses talk about caring as actions and behaviours. They may mention skills and procedures as proof of their caring actions for patients. Nurses speaking from within this discourse refer to caring using complex concepts such as providing comfort, showing compassion and helping others.

'Caring as knowing' is a discourse that contributes ideas and practices associated with the knowledge base essential for nursing. Nurses use statements in which they claim to own caring. Caring theorists have contributed much to this discourse (Leininger 1991; Orem 1991; Watson 1999; Watson et al 2002).

Consider the following questions.

- *Nursing is often called the caring profession. Is this how you view nursing?*
- *When observing the nurses you work with, what elements of their practice would you identify as caring and why?*
- *What would constitute uncaring practices by nurses?*

Coaching tips

- Reflect on the meaning of caring and identify what it means to you. Try to define caring. Identify how you demonstrate caring in your practice. Seek feedback about your practice from patients, peers and mentors. Does this feedback support your definitions and ideas about what caring is?
- Consider practices that may affect your clinical experience and your ability to undertake care; for example, the mix of staff on the ward or the model of care implemented.
- Compare your nursing practice with that of others. What similarities and differences are there?
- Consider your personality, philosophy and beliefs. How do these affect your caring practices?
- Consider the different types of practice experiences you undertake throughout your programme. Do you care differently for

patients in different practice contexts? Compare, for example, caring for people in a perioperative, emergency room or care home placement.

- Ask your patients for feedback about your practice. Ask specific questions: do they feel that you give them enough time, that you listen to them, and that you undertake nursing care in a timely manner?

4.2 Reflective practice

Something to think about...

Learning without thought is labour lost; thought without learning is perilous.

Confucius (551–479 BC), Chinese philosopher

At the risk of stating the obvious, simply undertaking a placement does not necessarily develop proficiency – just being there does not guarantee learning. Developing proficiency involves not only taking action in practice but also learning from practice through reflection. Reflection is intrinsic to learning. It allows nurses to process their experience, explore their understanding of what they are doing, why they are doing it, and what impact it has on themselves and others (Boud 1999; Peate 2006).

The skill of reflection is pivotal to the development of your clinical knowledge and understanding. Reflection allows you to consider your personal and professional skills, and to identify needs for ongoing development. As a student nurse you should become increasingly aware of your professional values, skills, strengths and areas that require further development.

Although we can and do learn from a wide range of experiences (good and bad), learning is often initiated by painful, difficult, embarrassing or uncomfortable experiences. Don't try just to forget about these challenging times. Reflection is about exploration, questioning, learning and growing through, and as a consequence of, these experiences.

Devoting some time to reflection during and after each practice experience will allow you to plan for future experiences and to develop clear and appropriate objectives for your next placement. At the very least, reflecting on your experience provides information that you can take to clinical or academic staff for help, or guidance, in further skill development.

Keeping a journal or reflective diary

The process of reflection provides the raw data of experiences. In order to use these experiences creatively, to transform them into knowledge, the additional stage of writing is required. Writing fixes thoughts on paper. As you stare at the paper, and stare at what you have written, your objectified thinking stares back at you. As you rearrange your writings, you often find that you are loosening your imagination by combining various ideas and thoughts. Creative ideas occur during the mechanical process of giving them shape (van Manen 1990). Reflections are the raw materials, but they are turned into knowledge as you write – sometimes you don't know how much you know until you write them down.

Many nursing programmes require students to participate in some form of formal written reflection. Students often have to write an assignment based on their reflections. Drawing upon ideas written in a reflective journal or diary will help in the recollection and ordering of your thoughts and help you to discuss your clinical experience, including application of relevant theory, and your understanding of that experience. Even if this is not a formal requirement at your educational institution, it is certainly wise to keep a personal account as the reflective writing process allows you to clarify your values, affirm your strengths and identify your learning needs.

Discerning and describing the knowledge, values and skills that go into day-to-day nursing work allow nurses to understand their work in a more empowering way. This increases nurses' mastery and appreciation of their own work and their ability to care better for patients (Buresh & Gordon 2000).

Something to think about...

Observation tells us the fact, reflection the meaning of the fact.
Florence Nightingale (in Baly 1991)

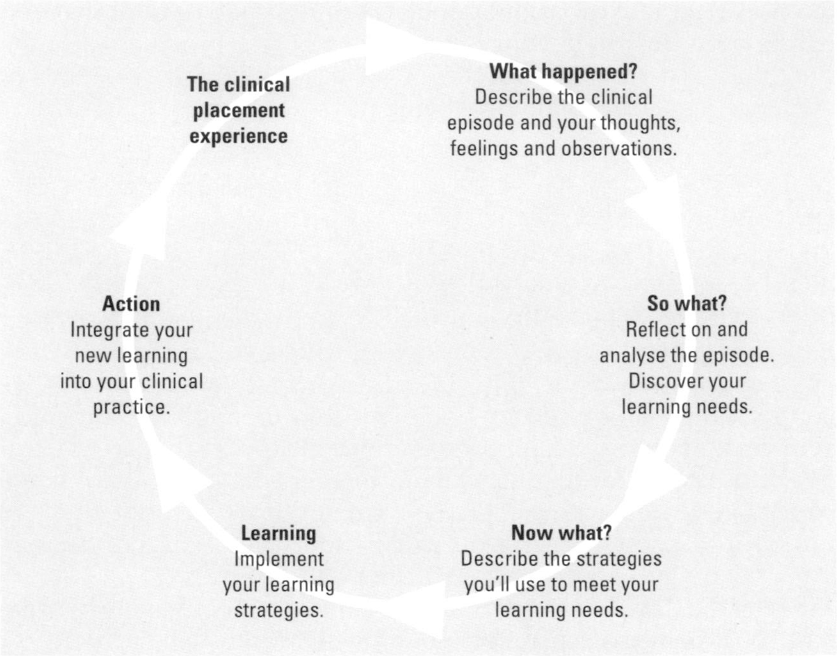

Figure 4.1   A reflective learning cycle. (Adapted from Driscoll 2000.)

Coaching tips

There are many resources to help you develop your ability to become a reflective practitioner, and your lecturers may recommend a process. Figure 4.1 is a diagrammatic representation of one method of reflection that many students find clear and easy to follow. Give it a try – you may be surprised how insightful you become!

4.3 Reality check and seeking feedback

So far in this book we have focused on the clinical environment and your place in it. Now it's time to turn the focus completely onto you, by asking you to address the following questions:

• How do I see myself?
• How do others see me?

This is not a once-off activity, but rather a lifelong process of personal and professional development. This 'reality check' is pivotal to your ongoing growth and improvement, and is a process that you will find invaluable to your career success.

How do I see myself?

To answer this question you should begin by assessing and listing your skills and attributes (clinical, interpersonal and others), and identifying your strengths and limitations. Skills are acquired abilities. Attributes may be acquired or intrinsic. There are three main types of skill and attribute:

- technical or clinical skills, such as those involved in providing oral care to an unconscious patient or safely administering medications
- interpersonal skills, which include communication, empathy and being supportive (among others)
- personal attributes, such as flexibility, resilience, self-efficacy, motivation, critical thinking and problem-solving.

Take some time to reflect on your skills and consider areas in which you excel and those that require further development. Identifying gaps or limitations is just as important as acknowledging your strengths.

How do others see me?

Once you have completed your self-assessment, you should validate it by seeking feedback from others. You can obtain this feedback from mentors, clinicians and fellow students. Performance appraisals and informal feedback are invaluable to understanding how others perceive you. Asking for feedback is not always easy, but your success depends on your openness to different perspectives. It involves listening and accepting positive and negative feedback, and acknowledging the areas in which change and improvement are needed. Seeking advice about new skills that you require and strategies to develop them is also essential.

Now compare the skills and attributes that you identified with the feedback from others. Are there any discrepancies? Did others recognize skills and attributes that you were not aware of but can now build on? Were limitations identified that you were not aware of?

> ## Something to think about...
>
> *If life is to have meaning, the extent to which you know yourself is the most important work that you will ever do. And because life is a process of emergence and becoming, it is a journey not a destination.*
>
> Crow (2000, p 33)

Coaching tips

It is your right (and responsibility) as a student to seek ongoing and regular feedback about your performance. Most educational institutions have a formal process for ensuring this occurs. However, you should still seek informal feedback regularly. Ask for specific, concrete feedback about your skills, attributes, strengths and limitations, and use the feedback as a springboard to success.

Lastly, receiving formal feedback should be a positive experience and should not display any hidden agendas, such as the discussion of any previously unmentioned problems. All problem areas – for example, poor time management skills or unsafe practice – should be dealt with when they occur and not stored up to be revealed only at a performance review. You deserve regular formative feedback throughout your clinical experience, and opportunities to improve. Grievance procedures are available if disagreements are unable to be resolved between you and your mentor, and you should consult your educational policies for guidance. Conflict and confusion, if they arise, should be dealt with constructively and sensitively.

4.4 Articulating your learning needs

> ## Something to think about...
>
> *Nurses are so hesitant to ask for what they need, they cannot accept the idea of asking for what they want. It seems too self indulgent.*
>
> Chenevert (1985, p 116)

In order to articulate your learning needs, you need to know what it is you require. Self-assessment is the key to exploring new opportunities (see Section 4.3). It will assist you to develop a list of needs that can then be articulated to mentors, teachers and other clinicians so that learning opportunities can be enhanced.

The following story illustrates one student's dilemma and highlights a case where articulation of the student's learning needs would have helped her to achieve her goals.

Hui Fei was undertaking her final practice experience. A component of this practice experience was her mentor's appraisal of her clinical performance. On two occasions during this experience, Hui Fei's mentor asked her whether she had any specific clinical skills for which she needed additional teaching, support or assessment. Hui Fei told her mentor that she was OK.

At the end of her practice experience period, Hui Fei produced her book for sign-off. At this point her mentor said that she could not complete several elements of the appraisal because she had not observed and assessed Hui Fei's practice across all the requisite areas. Naturally Hui Fei became upset, because she could not complete the requirements. Her mentor pointed out that she had asked her on more than one occasion if there was anything she needed to complete, and emphasized she could not sign off on areas that she had not observed.

In this scenario, the student did not articulate her needs to the mentor early in the placement, and on completion of the practice experience the expectations of the mentor and student were not congruent. Effective communication strategies are essential so that you can express your learning needs. As a student you are encouraged to identify your learning needs early in the practice experience, re-evaluating them as necessary.

Coaching tips

- Be prepared for each practice experience. Reflect on past experiences and your clinical strengths and weaknesses. Identify new learning appropriate for practice in the forthcoming placement environment.

- Find out about the opportunities available in the area of your practice experience to determine your personal objectives (before your arrival on the first day).
- When you introduce yourself to your mentor, request a time to discuss your learning objectives and assessment requirements.
- Ask your mentor for strategies to help you achieve your learning objectives.
- Find a quiet place at an appropriate time to discuss your needs with your mentor.
- Remember that questions during patient care episodes disrupt the therapeutic relationship and remove the focus from the patient. Be respectful of the patient and the need for the nurse to concentrate.

4.5 Ethical dilemmas in nursing

Something to think about...

You should not decide until you have heard what both have to say.
Aristophanes (Greek playwright, *c.*438 to *c.*388 BC), *The Wasps*

What is ethics and why do nurses need to understand it?

Ethics, also known as morality, is often defined as the philosophical study of right or wrong action (Dahnke & Dreher 2006). This does not mean that ethics is of concern to philosophers alone. All human beings have pondered questions of right and wrong from time to time. It is essential for nurses to understand ethics, because in their day-to-day work they frequently encounter ethical questions and problems such as a patient's rights, questions of life and death, and confidentiality. A clear understanding of ethics helps nurses to interpret these difficult situations and to identify possible courses of action and the principles underpinning moral actions (Dahnke & Dreher 2006).

Ethical principles

Ethical principles are standards of conduct that make up an ethical system.

Autonomy The ability to make free choices about oneself and one's life, to be self-governing. This principle is at the heart of informed consent.

Beneficence To do good, and the obligation to act for the benefit of others.

Non-maleficence To avoid doing harm.

Justice Fairness and the equal distribution of benefits and burdens.

(Adapted from Johnstone 2004.)

Which is more important, ethics or law?

This is a complicated question with no clear-cut answer. Law and ethics are not the same, but often overlap. Law describes the minimum standards of acceptable behaviour. Ethics describes the highest moral codes of behaviour.

What is an ethical dilemma?

A dilemma is defined as a problem where there is a choice to be made between options that seem equally unfavourable. A moral or ethical dilemma is even more complex. There may be conflicting moral principles that apply equally in a given situation, and neither can be chosen without violating the other.

Consider the case of a nurse who accepts the moral principle that demands sanctity of life, but who also accepts the moral principle of non-maleficence, which demands that people should be spared intolerable suffering. Imagine this nurse caring for a person who is terminally ill and suffering intolerable and intractable pain. In this situation, if the nurse accepts the sanctity-of-life principle, he or she would not be able to sanction the administration of the large and potentially lethal doses of narcotics that may be required to alleviate the patient's pain. On the other hand, if the principle of non-maleficence were followed, the nurse might

*be required to administer potentially lethal dose of narcotics, even though
this would probably hasten the patient's death.*

In this situation the nurse is confronted with a profound
dilemma. To uphold the sanctity-of-life principle would violate
the principle of non-maleficence, and to uphold the principle
of non-maleficence might violate the sanctity-of-life principle.
In everyday nursing practice, the nurse would be guided by
both principles; however, the ultimate question for the nurse
in this situation is 'Which ethical principle should I choose?'.
(Adapted from Johnstone 2004, p 51.)

---

*In another case, a nurse was caring for a patient from a traditional Greek
background who had been diagnosed with metastatic cancer. The doctor
had requested that the patient not be told his diagnosis.*

*However, the patient kept asking the nurse and his family for informa-
tion about his condition. The family knew the diagnosis, but wanted the
doctor to tell the patient. The nurse was caught between a duty to tell the
patient the truth as he was requesting (to promote the patient's right to
autonomy), and a duty to respect the family's wishes. The nurse was
also influenced by the expectation that the doctor's orders should be
followed.*

The question for the nurse in this situation is, again, 'Which
duty ought I to follow: my duty to the patient, to his family
or to the doctor?'. (Adapted from Johnstone 2004, pp
102–103.)

Ethics is a concept that you will undoubtedly study in your nursing
programme. You would be wise to consider and reflect upon ethical
situations as they arise in your nursing practice, being guided by
ethical principles and the Nursing and Midwifery Council (NMC)
Code of Professional Conduct (NMC 2008). Ethical dilemmas, when
they arise, may cause a great deal of distress and emotional turmoil.
In these situations, however, you are not alone and by communicating with your colleagues and mentors you will often find the support and guidance you need.

The incorporation of ethical principles into professional codes re-
inforces the nursing profession's intention to accept the rights of and
respect for individuals, and to uphold these in practice. The NMC Code
of Professional Conduct (NMC 2008) is complementary to the International Council of Nurses (2000) Code of Ethics for Nurses.

The purpose of codes based on ethical principles is to:

- identify the fundamental moral commitments of the profession
- provide nurses with a basis for professional and self-reflection on ethical conduct
- act as a guide to ethical practice
- indicate to the community the moral values that nurses can be expected to hold.

4.6 Crossing over the line

As a nursing student you will have many roles apart from that of a health professional. These roles may include neighbour, family member, friend and community member, among others. There may be times when the boundaries between your roles seem to blur. An example of this is when you become aware that one of the patients on your ward is someone you know. Nurses can find themselves in situations where professional boundaries are tested and they are expected to do the right thing according to their professional role (Peternelj-Taylor & Yonge 2003). Specific guidelines have established principles that must be adhered to, ensuring standards are met (NMC 2008; Scottish Executive 2004).

What are 'boundaries'?

Boundaries are limits to appropriate behaviour in our personal and professional relationships. Phrases such as 'crossing over the line' and 'overstepping the mark' are commonly used to describe inappropriate behaviour. In nursing these boundaries are linked to accountability, performance, conduct and ethics (NMC 2008).

What purpose do boundaries serve?

Maintaining appropriate boundaries in a nurse–patient relationship facilitates therapeutic practice and results in safe and effective care. On the one hand, nurses and nursing students may be too cold, distant or formal, so as to not be caring enough to be helpful, and, on the other hand, they may be overly involved, too interested, 'touchy–feely' or invasive. The creation of even a platonic relationship with a patient during a therapeutic relationship increases patient vulnerability, as does caring for a patient who you know from work, university/college or your community. There is a need to ensure that the nurse–patient therapeutic relationship is always conducted with the sole intent of benefiting the patient. Knowing the difference between a professional and a personal relationship, and being able to recognize boundaries between them, may seem like common sense. However, recognition of these boundaries requires knowledge and skills that are acquired through time and experience (Peternelj-Taylor & Yonge 2003). Consider the following situation.

A student nurse (James) was undertaking a clinical placement in a mental health unit when a fellow student (Jenny) was admitted following her attempted suicide. James did not know Jenny well but decided to call in and say hello to her. During the course of the next week James spent a lot of time with Jenny, believing his support to be therapeutic. Jenny opened up to him, sharing many details about her life. James began to disclose his own experiences of depression and how it was managed.

On return to university James happened to mention to some fellow students 'in confidence' that Jenny had been admitted to the mental health unit where he'd undertaken his practice experience. He hoped that they would be sensitive to the situation and understanding when Jenny returned to university. As often happens, 'news' spread and Jenny found out. She was devastated that James had broken her trust, even more so because she had shared so many sensitive details with him about her life. Jenny decided not to return to university. James was reported for misconduct.

Consider the implications of the above situation. The outcome could have been avoided if James had recognized and understood the NMC Code of Professional Conduct and considered his professional boundaries of practice. As a student, you may not have enough experience to guide your decisions. We suggest that you consult someone who has more experience.

Coaching tips

- Inform your mentor or ward sister immediately if you become aware of the presence of someone you know when on a practice experience.

- Refer to education and healthcare policies. Policy directives may mean that you are not to have direct responsibility for the care of a patient you know, or you may be requested to complete your placement in an alternative clinical area.
- Keep interactions with patients you know to a minimum.
- Remember always to maintain complete confidentiality regarding the admission and care of all patients, including people you know.
- Review Chapter 1, in which confidentiality is covered in more detail.

4.7 Punctuality and reliability

Punctuality and reliability are concepts often discussed in relation to work ethic. We need to consider what our ethics (or moral principles) are with regard to work, how these will be judged as good or bad, or right or wrong, and how they affect others.

Consider the following story. Although it does not focus specifically only on the student's role, the principles are nevertheless crucial to your understanding of professionalism.

Sandip was a student nurse who had been employed as a healthcare worker in operating theatres. At 7.15 a.m. after a long, tiring nightshift, Sandip was looking forward to having a rest. The night had seen multiple trauma cases come through into the emergency operating theatre unit. He had just received word that an accident had occurred in a nearby factory and several 'urgent' patients were on their way to the theatre. The dayshift staff would soon be on duty to care for these patients. Unfortunately, the person replacing Sandip had slept in. This meant that Sandip was required to stay back and work beyond his allocated shift. This had the potential to compromise patient and staff safety, as Sandip was tired.

The consequences of the nurse's sleep-in are several:

- Urgent care required by the patient is undertaken by tired night staff who are less able to concentrate after a long, busy shift.
- Staff relationships may be compromised when they are called upon to work longer hours. This could contribute to a reduction of tolerance in the work environment.

Coaching tips

- A good work ethic means that you are punctual for all shifts, meetings and appointments.
- Reflect upon your own practices and identify barriers that prevent you from being punctual.
- Be organized and prepare your uniform and other placement requirements in advance.
- Notify the appropriate person(s) if an untoward event occurs that prevents you from being on time.
- For new placements, trial and time the trip to the placement location (at the same time of the day, if possible).
- Allow plenty of time to get to the ward or unit, as there may be some distance to walk from the car park or public transport stop.

4.8 Taking the initiative

Something to think about...

As defined by the Oxford English Dictionary (2007), to initiate is to begin, to commence, and to take the initiative is to take the step or to lead into action.

Clinical experience is an integral and valuable component of student learning. Although clinical placements provide opportunities for students to develop clinical proficiency and to link theory with practice, students themselves must take the initiative to grow and learn during their placements.

Taking the initiative can be demonstrated in many ways, and students who show initiative are well regarded by team members. This leads to positive relationships between students and clinicians, in turn assisting student learning and contributing to increased confidence (Clare et al 2003).

Mentors and teachers expect students to achieve their learning objectives during their placement experiences. Inherent in this expectation is that students are self-directed and actively contribute to their own needs, making choices and decisions about learning (Reilly & Oermann 1992). Responsibility for learning therefore rests with students.

The following story shows how one student took the initiative.

Jolene always arrived early for practice experiences. When she arrived on this particular day, the clinicians were resuscitating a patient. Although Jolene wasn't scheduled to start her shift at this time, she suggested to the clinicians that she could assist by getting patients ready for breakfast, showering them and completing their observations. Jolene's action supported the clinicians while they were caring for a critical patient. Later they thanked Jolene for her initiative. Her contribution to the nursing team had ensured that all patients received ongoing care.

Jolene's story shows how initiative can result in a positive outcome. However, students do not always display initiative, as demonstrated by the following story.

Leo, a second-year nursing student, was allocated to a busy medical ward. On the third week of his practice experience, his mentor approached him about some of the problems that had been identified with his practice. Some of the issues were: Leo spent much of his time at the nurses' station rather than with his patients; he was missing from the ward on several occasions; and he had not showered the patients he had been asked to or made their beds.

Was Leo lacking in initiative? What may be the underlying issues for Leo? The discussion between Leo and his mentor highlights several perspectives. Leo said he was not confident in undertaking patient care. He admitted he had missed a number of his tutorials and lectures, and he was afraid to ask for help because he thought staff would see him as 'hopeless'. He was concerned that he would fail his placement because of this. He did not feel confident or comfortable and that is why he left the ward when he was asked to provide personal care to patients.

The clinical staff were concerned because Leo was not reliable and did not undertake nursing care as requested.

Coaching tips

- Be self-directed and ensure that you are thoroughly prepared for practice experiences.
- Seek out opportunities for learning by communicating well-thought-out clinical objectives that link theoretical learning with potential clinical opportunities.
- Be proactive in organizing your own clinical learning opportunities.
- Attend ward inservice sessions when available.

4.9 Putting work ahead of your studies

Clashes between work, study, practice experiences and personal commitments often cause problems for nursing students. Competing commitments can have an impact on your progress and achieving your goals. Thoughtful, advanced planning can prevent later problems. Be mindful that the effects of celebrations, fatigue, travel, illness, alcohol and drugs may lead you to be unproductive on placement rather than motivated and committed to learn. Consider Lara's story.

Lara was in her third and final year of the nursing programme and was also working at her local hospital as a healthcare worker. She worked Friday, Saturday and Sunday nights routinely and sometimes picked up other shifts during holiday periods. Lara felt pressured at times to undertake additional shifts. She wanted to be seen as interested, motivated and hard working, and was keen to secure a position there as a registered nurse when she qualified. She did not discuss her roster with the sister in charge, even though Lara knew that she was due to commence a full-time placement. She continued to work her routine hours and added additional shifts when requested.

During Lara's placement, the mentor informed her tutor that Lara was performing adequately, but because Lara's apparent tiredness was of concern it had been decided not to ask her to care for any complex patients, or to undertake any advanced skills. She was not permitted to administer medication and was allocated showering, feeding and bed-making only. Kate's mentor felt that it was not safe for her to perform care commensurate with her educational level.

Further discussions between the mentor and the tutor revealed that Lara had already been sent home on the previous day because she was tired.

When she had admitted that she had worked the previous nightshift, she had been sent home for safety reasons.

In the above scenario, what issues can be identified?

- Patient safety is the most important issue that needs to be considered. Lara has a responsibility to undertake care to the level of her knowledge in a safe, accountable manner. Her tiredness detracted from her ability to perform safely.
- Educational institutions have in place policies that guide student behaviour, both in the classroom and on placements. At Lara's institution, her behaviour contravened those policies, and negatively affected her progress in her nursing programme.

It is important to maintain a 'life in balance'; this includes your biological, psychological, sociocultural, environmental and politicoeconomic health (Holland et al 2008). Allow time for study and make thoughtful decisions about where your energy is to be spent. You must be at 'full capacity' on practice experience to ensure that you provide safe nursing care and can learn effectively.

Coaching tips

- Be accountable, safe and responsible for all practice undertaken.
- Plan all activities in advance and avoid clashes between work, other commitments and clinical learning experiences.
- Prioritize and organize your life.

Activity

Investigate the student support services that are available at your educational and healthcare institutions. Identify how these services can be of support to you during practice experience.

Reflective thinking activities

Self-assessment

Complete this self-assessment to help you understand who you are and what is important to you as a nurse.

What types of placements have I most preferred? Why?

(e.g. I preferred experiences that were not fast paced. I had time to sit and talk to my patients and I felt I could ask lots of questions because the staff were not rushed.)

_____

_____

_____

What types of placement have I least preferred? Why?

(e.g. I sometimes felt overwhelmed in the fast-paced, highly technical experiences, and did not always feel I could contribute.)

_____

_____

_____

What motivates and inspires me to be the best nurse I can be?

(e.g. Good role models who are skilled, knowledgeable and excited to be nurses; positive feedback from other nurses and patients.)

_____

_____

_____

What is most important to me when I am nursing?

(e.g. Learning something new every day; knowing I've made a difference in one person's life; feeling part of the nursing team.)

_____

_____

_____

I made a difference on a placement when ...

(e.g. I was able to advocate for a patient who was in a lot of pain, so that a different type of analgesia was ordered for him.)

_____

_____

_____

My greatest strengths as a nurse are ...

(e.g. Eagerness and motivation; communication skills with staff and patients.)

_____

_____

_____

My limitations as a nurse are ...

(e.g. Not enough confidence to challenge nursing care that is not best practice; documentation; patient assessment skills.)

_____

_____

_____

Reality check

What type of feedback have I received from patients, nursing staff and my mentors about my strengths?

_____

_____

_____

What type of feedback have I received from patients, nursing staff and my mentors about my limitations?

_____

_____

_____

How did my self-assessment compare with others' assessment of me?

_____

_____

_____

What will I do to enhance my strengths and address my limitations? (Be very realistic and strategic.)

_____

_____

_____

Whose support and guidance do I need to help me enhance my strengths and address my limitations?

_____

_____

_____

References

Baly M (ed.) 1991 As Miss Nightingale said. Scutari Press, London

Boud D 1999 Avoiding the traps: seeking good practice in the use of self-assessment and reflection in professional courses. Social Work Education 18(2): 121–132

Bourgeois S 2006 An archive of caring for nursing. PhD thesis, University of Western Sydney, Penrith

Buresh B, Gordon S 2000 From silence to voice. What nurses know and must communicate to the public. Cornell University Press, New York

Chenevert M 1985 Pro-nurse handbook. Designed for the nurse who wants to thrive professionally. Mosby, St Louis

Clare J, Brown D, Edwards H et al 2003 Evaluating clinical learning environments: creating education–practice partnerships and clinical education benchmarks for nursing. Learning outcomes and curriculum development in major disciplines: Nursing phase 2 final report. School of Nursing and Midwifery, Flinders University, Adelaide

Crow G L 2000 Knowing self. In: Bower F L (ed.). Nurses taking the lead: personal qualities of effective leadership. WB Saunders, Philadelphia, p 15–37

Dahnke M, Dreher M 2006 Defining ethics and applying theories. In: Lachman V (ed.). Applied ethics in nursing. Springer, New York, p 3–13

Driscoll J 2000 Practising clinical supervision. A reflective approach. Baillière Tindall, Edinburgh

Holland K, Jenkins J, Solomon J, Whittam S 2008 Applying the Roper Logan Tierney model in practice. Churchill Livingstone, Elsevier, Edinburgh

International Council of Nurses 2000 Code of ethics for nurses. International Council of Nurses, Geneva

Johnstone M 2004 Bioethics: a nursing perspective, 4th edn. Churchill Livingstone, Sydney

Leininger M M 1991 The theory of culture care diversality and universality. In: Leininger M M (ed.). Culture care diversity and universality: a theory of nursing. National League for Nursing, New York, p 5–68

Nursing and Midwifery Council 2008 The NMC code of professional conduct: standards of conduct, performance and ethics for nurses and midwives. Online. Available: http://www.nmc-uk.org/aFrameDisplay.aspx?DocumentID=3954 6 June 2008

Orem D 1991 Nursing concepts of practice, 3rd edn. McGraw-Hill, New York

Oxford English Dictionary 2007 Online. Available: http://dictionary.oed.com 24 Aug 2007

Peate I 2006 Becoming a nurse in the 21st century. John Wiley, Chichester

Peternelj-Taylor C A, Yonge O 2003 Exploring boundaries in the nurse–client relationship: professional roles and responsibilities. Perspectives in Psychiatric Care 39(2): 55–66

Reilly D E, Oermann M H 1992 Clinical teaching in nursing education. National League for Nursing, New York

Scottish Executive 2004 Framework for nursing in general practice. Online. Available: http://www.scotland.gov.uk/publications/2004/09/19966/43294 24 Aug 2007

van Manen M 1990 Researching lived experience. State University of New York Press, New York

Walsh M, Walsh A 1999 Measuring patient satisfaction with nursing care: experience using the Newcastle satisfaction with nursing scale. Journal of Advanced Nursing 29(2):307–315

Watson J 1999 Postmodern nursing and beyond. Churchill Livingstone, Edinburgh

Watson R, Stimpson A Topping A et al 2002 Clinical competence assessment in nursing: a systematic review of the literature. Journal of Advanced Nursing 39(5): 421–431

Williams A M 1998 The delivery of quality nursing care: a grounded theory study of the nurse's perspective. Journal of Advanced Nursing 27: 808–816

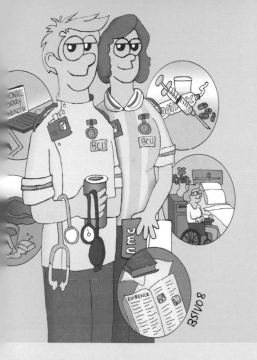

Chapter 5

How you communicate

Envision how things would be if the voice and visibility of nursing were commensurate with the size and importance of nursing in health care.

Buresh & Gordon (2000, p 11)

Introduction

This chapter will help to add another layer of knowledge, skills and insight to your repertoire of clinical attributes. It describes how you can make meaningful contributions to the clinical environment through sensitive attention to the way you communicate with patients and peers. In the first section we also describe the ways in which nurses can exercise their power to define and promote their profession by effectively using their 'nursing voice'.

5.1 What is a nurse?

In this section we draw from the work of Bernice Buresh and Suzanne Gordon, two journalists who have written extensively on the importance of nurses being able to define and promote their profession.

The public holds nurses in very high regard. Opinion polls indicate that nurses are the most highly rated profession in terms of honesty and ethics, rating significantly higher than pharmacists, teachers or doctors. Yet studies indicate that when people think of registered nurses they are more inclined to dwell on their kindness and caring than on their knowledge, expertise or professionalism. The public's awareness of nurses' professionalism is linked to nurses' ability to highlight their experience, skills and expertise.

The job at hand for nurses is to help the public (as well as other healthcare professionals) to construct an authentic meaning of the word 'nurse' that conveys the richness and uniqueness of nursing. This means not misconstruing nursing as something commonplace, but deepening the public's comprehension of nursing as deeply complex, skilled and essential to patient care (adapted from Buresh & Gordon 2000, p 17).

Coaching tips

How do you introduce yourself?
Nurses have a choice about the way they present themselves to patients, families, doctors, other clinicians and the general public. They can present themselves in ways that assert their personal and professional identity, or they can remain part of the wider, undifferentiated healthcare services industry. They can highlight their clinical knowledge and proficiency, or they can conceal it. Each day in the workplace, what nurses say and do can elicit the respect and collegial treatment their professional standing deserves, or undermine it. While caring for patients and families, or interacting with other members of the healthcare team, nurses convey messages about their own respect for the status of nursing. Some of these messages are implicit; others are more explicit, delivered through presentation, body language, tone of voice and conversational style.

Some examples to think about. . .

If a nurse thinks it advisable to consult a doctor, she or he can inform the patient by saying, 'I'll discuss this with the doctor'. By using these words, nurses imply that they have clinical knowledge and judgement, and see themselves as doctors' colleagues. Alternatively nurses can act in a subservient way by saying, 'I'll have to ask the doctor'.

When contacting a doctor, a nurse can establish collegiality by beginning the conversation with the words, 'Hello, Dr Smith. This is Sarah O'Shea (or Nurse O'Shea), Mrs Johnson's nurse. She is experiencing chest pain and I think ...'. Alternatively, she can cast herself in an inferior role by beginning, 'I'm so sorry to bother you Dr Smith, but this is Sarah, Mrs Johnson's nurse ...'.

The way that nurses introduce themselves to patients and their families can also have a significant impact on how they are perceived. You can introduce yourself with a firm handshake, provide your full name, inform them that you are a student nurse and explain your role in the patient's care. Or you can simply say, 'Hello, I'm John' and leave it at that.

Most patients meeting you for the first time have few visual cues about your identity and role. Your introduction is your best opportunity to let people know that you are a student nurse, a serious professional with clinical skills and knowledge. Being serious and professional is not the same as being distant and aloof. It simply means presenting yourself as a knowledgeable caregiver. This presentation tends to reassure patients rather than alienate them.

First name basis?

It has become increasingly common for nurses to use only their first names when introducing themselves to patients, visitors or doctors. Even some name badges bear only first names. Although society has become more informal, few doctors introduce themselves by their first names? Why then is there an imbalance between these two professions? If nurses continue to uphold and reinforce these identification practices, it suggests that nurses regard doctors as superior in the healthcare environment. We know that this is not the real intention of nurses who use only their first names. Mostly they are doing it to develop a friendly and informal relationship with their patients, and to show them that they are 'on their side' or 'an equal'. Unfortunately, this often misconstrues what patients really want and need from a nurse. They don't want a friend: they want a nurse with knowledge and skill. 'A really good nurse will establish the context for a relationship. They will communicate to a patient: This is what I do. This is what you do. This is what I know. I will make sure that everything will be all right for you' (Buresh & Gordon 2000, p 52).

5.2 Welcome to the UK

This section is related to the topic of cultural competence discussed in Chapter 3. It is written especially for international students, although it will undoubtedly be of benefit to local students who want better to understand and support their peers. We hope that this brief overview will complement what you learn in class about contemporary practice cultures in the UK and help you to become accustomed to the clinical learning environment and the diverse factors that affect your learning experience. Without this knowledge, miscommunication is common and learning possibilities sometimes reduced.

Firstly, and most importantly, we'd like to say welcome to the UK. Having international students in academic programmes such as nursing has had a positive impact on our ability to appreciate and understand different cultures. The diversity and richness that you bring to the academic and clinical environment enhances the learning opportunities of all students and staff.

Although most students will at some stage experience difficulties related to their clinical placement, these may be exacerbated by language and cultural differences. If you experience problems, it is important to reflect upon, try to distinguish and analyse the root cause of the problems so that appropriate support, guidance and teaching can be provided. Try to identify your fundamental issues of concern from the coaching tips below (adapted from Remedios & Webb 2005).

Coaching tips

Receptive communication (verbal and non-verbal)
Do you sometimes find it hard to understand what your patients or nursing colleagues are saying to you? Local accents, shortened, fast speech and the use of colloquialisms may cause significant difficulties for international students. Misunderstandings between you and others may occur if you do not readily acknowledge when you have not understood or have only partially understood a conversation. Most importantly, patients' safety may be jeopardized if you are not perfectly clear about what is being asked of you. Initially it may be culturally difficult for you to do this, but keep in mind that in the UK it is

not considered disrespectful to ask someone to repeat what they have said. Nor is it considered a 'failure' on your part if you have not understood something. On the contrary, clinicians will expect you to ask questions, and to ask for clarification whenever you need to.

Strategies for improvement
- If you want to confirm your understanding of an instruction or discussion, try paraphrasing: for example, 'Can I confirm that you'd like me to take Mrs Smith to the shower on a commode, because of her low blood pressure?'.
- Ask others to explain any colloquial language you do not understand.
- If you are unsure of healthcare terminology related to the patient mix on the ward where you are undertaking your placement, ask questions and be prepared to do some research.
- Remember, nodding or silence following a conversation may be taken to indicate that you fully understood what was being said, even if the reverse is true.

Expressive communication (verbal and non-verbal)
Do you sometimes find it difficult and frustrating trying to make yourself understood by patients or nursing colleagues? In the UK, you will be expected to be fluent in the English language, familiar with colloquialisms, and conversant with the professional language used for reporting and communicating with health professionals, but still have the ability to switch to less formal language when needed, for example when conversing with patients.

Strategies for improvement
- Observing nursing staff communicating effectively with one another and with patients will allow you to compare this with what you are used to, help you clarify expectations and enable you to build upon what you already know.
- Reflect on these observations carefully. Ask yourself what made the interactions effective. How and why was humour used? What colloquialisms and terms need clarification?
- Make the most of opportunities to practise communicating with patients and staff.
- Do not hesitate to ask your mentor to observe you and provide detailed feedback on your progress.

- Most educational institutions have student support services that provide English-language tuition. Avail yourself of this opportunity if you require additional help.

Written communication

Is it sometimes difficult to understand what is written or to find the English words for what you want to write? Both international and local students can experience difficulties with reading and writing. Patients' notes, referral letters, medication charts and other forms of professional documentation may be especially problematic as students try to find and use appropriate language and grammar.

Strategies for improvement

- Practise, practise, practise! Try writing a nursing report on notepaper and asking someone you respect and trust to critique it for you before you write in a patient's notes.
- Reading nursing journals will help you to develop your fluency in English and your professional vocabulary, and will build on what you already know.
- Even reading good-quality English-language novels will improve your literacy and grammar, and help you to understand better colloquialisms and local culture. Ask your librarian to recommend appropriate novels.
- Remember that in nursing reports you must always sign your name in English.

Cultural issues

Are you finding the clinical culture in the UK confusing and stressful? If you have no previous experience with Western healthcare systems, it will be difficult at first to understand the complexity of the structures and values operating within the system. The interactions between you and patients or fellow students may present unique problems. This applies not only to international students but also to local students caring for patients from diverse cultures. Misunderstandings may involve religion, gender and age-related issues, as well as language. Sometimes the lack of understanding and tolerance on the part of clinical staff and fellow students may have a negative impact on the ability of international students to fit into and feel accepted in the clinical environment.

Strategies for improving understanding

- Many educational institutions have dedicated courses or at least an orientation programme to prepare students for the cultural differences they may encounter. Local colleges may also provide programmes to assist with reading, writing and speaking. Make the most of these learning opportunities as well as the opportunities to interact with local students.
- Join local sporting, musical or recreational clubs to increase your opportunities for socializing with people from different backgrounds.
- During your clinical placement experience it is important that you express any concerns you have, even though it may be difficult to do so. Sharing your worries with someone you trust will mean that you can be supported and guided. Sadly, not all students, staff or patients will be sensitive to different health beliefs, customs, and cultural and religious practices. If you experience discrimination, subtle or obvious, you need to discuss it with your educator or academic staff member. All educational and healthcare institutions in the UK have policies regarding discrimination, and your concerns will be taken seriously.
- Seek out a peer mentor to work with during your studies. This should be a person who can support your development in the English language. Spend time together focusing on language development and understanding.
- 'Everyday English for nursing' (Grice 2003) is an excellent resource to help you develop your English language skills.

5.3 Using professional language

Nurses must be able to describe the care they give and the clinical decisions they make (Buresh & Gordon 2000). In discussions with colleagues, patients, their significant others and the public, the language that nurses use reflects on their professional standing. Nursing students are recognized as a part of this group of professionals and are expected to behave according to the conventions of the nursing profession.

You will accumulate professional and jargon-based words and statements that will become a normal part of your practice language. Nursing jargon refers to words that are used by nurses when they talk about their practice. These words may exclude people who are unfamiliar with their use, so choose your words carefully when you speak to people who do not have a nursing background. Distinguish between what you say to health workers and what you say to the lay person (Buresh & Gordon 2000). Colloquial language, or slang, is often referred to as conversational speech without constraint. While appropriate perhaps in some contexts, its use should be minimized in the practice environment.

For some nurses, it is not unusual for them to address their patients, particularly if they are elderly, using an endearment (sweetie, cherub, darling, angel, lovey, etc.) (Gardner et al 2001). However, many patients will be offended by being addressed in this manner, so don't assume that it is acceptable. A good rule is to simply ask your patient whether they would prefer you to use their given name (e.g. John) or address him more formally (Mr Smith).

As you progress through your nursing programme you will develop a wide repertoire of professional terminology. Give careful consideration to your audience to ensure that you use the most appropriate language in each situation. Nursing terminology and medical terms are words that should not be confused. Their inappropriate use will completely change the meaning of your message. Abbreviations must be approved by the institution in which you are undertaking your placement. Some words that are commonly abbreviated can have very different meanings within various contexts of practice.

Coaching tips

- Reflect upon language used in professional situations and how it affects others.
- Take stock of the language you use: words, selected statements (informal and formal), tone and loudness.
- Consider who you are speaking to and their age, culture, medical condition, status and knowledge.
- Consider the words, statements and conventions of language that are appropriate in each situation.
- Select words that cannot easily be misinterpreted.
- Explain medical and nursing terms to patients using language that is easily understood.
- Be aware that the way in which a word is interpreted may be influenced by thoughts, feelings and beliefs that people may have about that word (e.g. drug versus medication, or miscarriage versus abortion).

- Avoid the use of colloquial and coarse language in the practice environment (many people are offended by swearing).
- Consider the effect of words on others (some words may convey a false sense of urgency to a patient).
- Learn the meaning of medical terminology and use the terms accurately (e.g. words ending in -ectomy, -ology, -oscopy, -otomy, etc.).
- Make a list of accepted abbreviations.
- Listen to the way your role model uses professional language.
- Consider that the use of certain words may offend, alienate or detract from your intended meaning.

5.4 Patient handover

The patient handover report is a communication practice used by nurses and other allied health carers to communicate nursing care requirements, patients' conditions and progress at change of shift. The purpose of nursing reports (handover) is to provide continuity of care amongst nurses. These reports may be given verbally in person, taped or written (Potter & Perry 2005).

In some institutions handovers may be undertaken at patient rounds, with patients and their families also contributing to decision-making and care-planning. In others, handovers may be held in the staff room or nurses' station, with nurses from the previous shift joined by nurses for the next shift. In these situations, the handover time is an opportunity for nurses to come together to discuss patient care as a team. Because of time constraints, reports are sometimes taped. The advantage of taping is that nurses can provide their handover at a convenient time during the shift, although this does not allow nurses to clarify and review care as they would in a face-to-face handover.

Change-of-shift reports should be conducted efficiently to enable one group to leave and the other group to begin the shift. The handover report describes the health status of patients, any aberrations from normal, interventions implemented and the effectiveness of interventions (such as analgesia). Information needs to be accurate, objective, concise, logical and to the point.

It is important for students to make the most of opportunities to be present at patient handover reports. Practise giving and receiving handover about your patient's condition and care requirements. Ask your mentor for advice and feedback about your handover.

Coaching tips

- Be on time for shift handover and remain for the entire process.
- Take notes and ask questions about anything you are unsure of.
- Be respectful of the people you are discussing. Avoid the use of judgemental language, and do not label or stereotype your patients or make negative comments about them.
- Use correct terminology, professional language, and only easily understood and recognized abbreviations.
- Avoid repetition and irrelevant data.
- Discuss with your mentor issues that need clarification.

5.5 Your voice in the clinical environment

Your voice is one of your most effective communication tools. You should be aware how you use this tool, and make it an efficient mechanism in your repertoire of skills. Reflect upon the pitch and tone of your voice so that you are aware of how you come across to others. The following are some extreme examples:

- calling down the corridor
- speaking so quietly that patients cannot hear what is being said to them
- a group of nurses laughing loudly at the nurses' station.

Clinical environments are different in structure and design. They can be small, intimate rooms where patients are interviewed, or rooms attached to a long corridor. Corridors echo, and the sound of people's voices can carry over long distances and traverse hard surfaces such as doors and walls. A comment made to a patient in one room may be very appropriate, but if the comment is overheard in an adjoining room it may unnecessarily frighten or distress someone. Think carefully about the pitch of your voice when talking to others.

Pitch of voice is critical to the development of appropriate communication skills. A loud voice is easily heard, but also easily overheard. Some people find that their voice projects well and that other people have no trouble hearing what they say. People with this type of voice need to be mindful of how far their voice carries. If you are aware that you have a loud voice, try standing next to the person you are talking to rather than speaking from a distance. This technique has the effect of reducing the projection factor you add to your voice when speaking at a distance (even short distances). Use eye contact to help direct your voice.

On the other hand, a soft voice can be difficult to hear and detracts from the message being conveyed. It can be a source of frustration for the listener. If you have a very soft voice, remember that any physical barriers (such as masks or curtains around a bed) may render your voice difficult to hear. Keep what you say clear, simple and straightforward. Connect with those to whom you are speaking to engage their attention (maintain eye contact, position yourself, use appropriate gestures). Practise voice projection to enable your voice to be heard within a group. Move forward in a group to engage people in the conversation so that you are speaking within a closer range.

Accents have a powerful effect on the listener's ability to understand what is being said. If you speak with an accent that is unfamiliar to those you are working with, you may need to slow your speech to allow the listener to 'attune' to the accent initially so that communication is effective.

Coaching tips

- Assess your voice – is it too loud or too soft for effective communication? Try taping yourself and then listening to the tape. Ask family or friends to give you some feedback about how you sound.
- Walk up to people to communicate rather than using a broadcast format.
- Consider the number of people that need to hear you and the type of information that it is important to convey. Reflect upon the situation and modify your voice to suit.
- Be aware of how you sound during spoken communication practices. Is your voice squeaky, high-pitched, growling or guttural?
- Consider how fast or slowly you speak, and the associated pitch of your voice.
- Be careful of how your voice projects in long corridors or large rooms.
- If you are concerned about your voice and the impact it has on others, seek feedback, and try to improve your speech by attending training sessions or public speaking groups.

5.6 Telephones and the internet

The use of telephones and the internet as communication tools in modern society has progressed rapidly. Both forms of communication are certainly convenient, but they can also be intrusive and annoying. Because telephones and the internet are essential for workplace communication, there are some guidelines that you should be aware of.

Most clinical facilities have policies that govern the use of telephones and the internet. Ward or unit telephones and computers are the property of the healthcare institution, and financial costs are associated with their use. Unless it is essential for you to make a personal phone call or to send an urgent email, remember that the telephones and computers are for business use only. Using a telephone for personal calls may prevent other healthcare staff from using it to give or receive information relevant to patient care. Similarly, spending time on the ward computer prevents others from using it for more important patient care purposes.

When you start on each new ward, ask what the policies are regarding telephone and internet access. In some facilities students are not to answer telephones or to give out patient information, and in many situations internet access is restricted to staff only.

Telephone etiquette

When you use the telephone you will be expected to use appropriate telephone etiquette.

- Answer the telephone promptly.
- Begin the conversation with your location, name and designation.
- Discontinue any conversation or activity before answering the telephone (such as eating, typing, etc.).
- Speak clearly and distinctly, using a pleasant tone of voice.
- Inform the caller when you are putting them on 'hold', and press the 'hold' button, so they do not overhear other conversations that may be held at the nursing station.
- Tell callers what your actions will be before you undertake them (e.g. I am going to transfer you to another number).
- Always be courteous, friendly and ready to assist the caller.
- Pass on messages promptly – it is best to write the messages down rather than rely on your memory.

The use of mobile phones

A mobile phone is now far more than just a telephone and is often referred to as a multi-media device with wireless connectivity. In the clinical learning environment a mobile phone has the potential to cause interference with technological equipment, and some healthcare institutions may request you to turn it off as you enter.

Your use of mobile phones during placement needs to be considered carefully. Making and receiving calls or text messaging should be done only in your breaks, and if urgent.

You should also take care when using your phone as a multi-media device. Consider the following scenario.

Nikos had been allocated to the special care nursery for his practice experience. He was very excited and enthusiastic about this placement, as it was an area that he wanted to work in once qualified. During the course of his placement, Nikos came across a baby who had a severe birth deformity. To help him to remember the condition, he took a series of photos using his mobile phone, so that he could develop a learning portfolio.

At his debrief session, Nikos shared his learning ideas with the other students and his clinical educator. Nikos had not sought written consent for the photos of the baby, and by using his mobile phone in this way he had unknowingly contravened the educational and healthcare institutions' policies.

Here are some other instances of where phones have been used inappropriately:

- text messaging friends during the handover report
- listening to music on a mobile while carrying out patient care
- booking football tickets while waiting for a patient to finish in the bathroom.

Coaching tips

- Develop courteous and effective telephone etiquette. Speak clearly and not too fast.
- Be mindful of the type of information you can divulge over the telephone in your role as a student, and to whom.
- Always find out details about the person you are speaking to at the beginning of the call.

- Know the protocols for taking patient care orders, test results and medication prescriptions over the phone and adhere to these conventions strictly.
- Know the healthcare facility's protocols for speaking to the media or the police.
- Always put the principles of confidentiality and privacy into practice when answering telephones during placement.
- When phoning a doctor, be organized. Have the information about the patient ready so that you can answer any questions. Make sure you are aware of the patient's clinical condition, recent vital signs and other assessments before you make the call.
- Make phone calls on your mobile phone and check for voice and text messages only in your breaks.
- Leave your placement location details (ward phone number) with your significant other in case of an emergency.
- Keep the contact details up to date in your student record – telephone and email are often used by lecturers to contact you to clarify learning issues.
- Access the internet only for patient care or educational purposes and with the permission of the appropriate staff.

Telephone order guidelines

- Clarify any telephone orders given by a doctor.
- Confirm the name of the patient at the beginning of the call.
- Repeat any orders back to the medical officer.
- Where required, a second person should listen to and countersign the order.
- Record the complete order in the patient's notes, including the date and time of the call, and the medical officer's name.

5.7 Self-disclosure

Self-disclosure is an act of revelation. What should you reveal about yourself in the course of your practice experience and to whom? Should you share your medical history or problems with your clients?

Some practice experiences provide the opportunity for you to attend group meetings. During these meetings, clients often disclose personal information about themselves and at times you may be tempted to share your experiences about a similar problem. Be cautious! The invitation by the group leader to be a part of the group is in your capacity as a nursing student. It is not for you to discuss your personal circumstances, conditions or history. The intention is for you to learn from the global concepts illustrated in the group discussions and to focus on the therapeutic interactions that occur. In group meetings, attention should not be drawn away from clients.

The same principles apply if you have the opportunity to be involved in a case conference. Objective, informed discussion that focuses on the clients is the purpose of the meetings. Don't be tempted to disclose personal information about yourself, even if it seems relevant.

Although there may be a few instances in which self-disclosure may be appropriate, it should always be well thought out and never be done to satisfy your own needs (e.g. as a medical consultation or to gain sympathy). Before you engage in self-disclosure, reflect on your own agenda and motivation. Is your self-disclosure a genuine act to help others or a way to satisfy your own needs?

Coaching tips

- Before you join a group counselling session, seek guidelines from the group leader about your role in group meetings.
- Monitor your behaviour to ensure that you do not take attention away from members of the group (for example, continually swishing your hair, sighing, moving around the room).
- Show respect and listen attentively to members of the group.
- Arrive on time for the group session and wait until the end to leave.
- Avoid talking to fellow students during a group therapy session. The focus is on the patients, and short conversations with a colleague are viewed as disrespectful and can often make patients or other group members angry.
- Do not at any time disclose any personal information. This includes your medical or psychological history (and any other history you may have).

- Save questions until after the meeting – it is not a question and answer session.
- Always thank the group members for allowing you to participate in their session.

5.8 Providing effective feedback

Feedback is an important component of student learning during practice experiences. It contributes to ongoing improvement when supported by quality feedback mechanisms. Feedback has the power to motivate others and to facilitate change and learning.

The concept of feedback is complex. It provides information about past performance and provides strategies for future learning. The degree to which feedback facilitates change, learning and future performance depends on many factors, including the perception and acceptance of the feedback by the recipient, the way feedback is conveyed, and the personal characteristics of persons involved.

Feedback should not be viewed as a bureaucratic process or a tool for control. It is not about being punitive, but offers a mechanism to enhance communication and teamwork. It is a powerful motivator for change. Effective feedback provides the potential to increase self-esteem and workplace satisfaction.

Mechanisms for providing feedback may be formal or informal (Penman & Oliver 2004). Formal feedback mechanisms may be hard-copy or online questionnaires that incorporate a rating scale, or forms that request open-ended comments. While you may receive feedback about your clinical performance, you may also be requested to give feedback about your clinical experiences or your mentor. Your feedback needs to be considered carefully, given freely, and with the intent to inform and to be honest. For feedback to be most effective, it should be provided immediately after your practice experience, so that you capture your thoughts, feelings and ideas. You have the right to question whether privacy and confidentiality principles are operational. Informal and spontaneous feedback is also a valuable mechanism to affirm and value others. Do not be afraid to offer constructive feedback during your learning experiences.

Feedback on student performance

You should also expect to receive regular feedback from the nurses you work with and your mentor. This may be in the form of a formal evaluation of your clinical performance or as opportunistic feedback that provides you with immediate information about your performance of a specific task or situation.

Feedback needs to be given in an environment conducive to listening and comprehending (quiet and away from the distraction of other people), and at a time when you can pay attention to what is being said. Your willingness to accept and to respond to the feedback is an important factor in the feedback process. Listen attentively, reflect on what is said, and be willing to discuss the issues presented. Negotiation and assertiveness skills will allow you to seek and qualify information. Ask for examples to illustrate a particular criterion. Show how you have learnt from situations and moved forward in your learning during the session. Be proactive and ask for strategies that will help you develop further. Your feedback session is not the time to bring up complaints about individuals. Issues of this kind should be dealt with at the time they occur. Most institutions have a mechanism for handling complaints or for commending someone.

Coaching tips

- Take every opportunity to provide feedback and to support quality mechanisms and processes. Remember that your feedback has the power to change practices and is therefore a critical component of your professional life.
- Make constructive comments when providing feedback.
- Mention a positive comment before a negative one.
- Take time to reflect upon your feedback before you submit it.
- Be receptive to feedback about your performance. Actively strive to grow and develop from constructively offered feedback.

Reflective thinking activities

How do you introduce yourself to staff on the first day of a clinical placement?

_____

_____

_____

How do you introduce yourself to your patients when you first meet them?

_____

_____

_____

You are a third-year student. One of the patients you have been caring for is febrile (38.7°C), oxygen saturation level is 89% and respiratory rate is 34. The registered nurse you are working with is tied up and asks you to phone the doctor. How do you prepare for the phone call and what will you say to the doctor?

_____

_____

_____

Tape yourself giving a simulated patient handover, then critique yourself.

1. What are your impressions of both the content of the handover, the way it was delivered and the way it sounded? Did you focus on the most important aspects of the patient's condition and care? If not, why not?

_____

_____

_____

2. Did you use the correct terminology? Give examples.

_____

_____

_____

3. Did you sound confident or timid? How can you improve this?

_____

_____

_____

_____

4. Was your voice clear and articulate, or did you mumble and stumble over your words?

_____

_____

_____

5. Were you too loud, too soft or too monotone?

_____

_____

_____

Imagine it is the last day of your clinical placement. You have had some great times there with some wonderful and supportive staff. However, you have also worked with a few registered nurses who made it obvious to you that they resented students. They were dismissive of your questions and unappreciative of your help. Write a letter to the ward sister about your experiences in the unit.

References

Buresh B, Gordon S 2000 From silence to voice. What nurses know and must communicate to the public. Cornell University Press, New York

Gardner A, Goodsell J, Duggan T, Murtha B, Peck C, Williams J 2001 'Don't call me sweetie'. Collegian 8(3):32–38

Grice T 2003 Everyday English for nursing. Elsevier, Edinburgh

Penman J, Oliver M 2004 Meeting the challenges of assessing clinical placement venues in a Bachelor of Nursing program. Online. Available: http://jutlp.uow.edu.au/2004_v01_i02/penman002.html 11 Jan 2005

Potter P, Perry A (eds) 2005 Fundamentals of nursing, 6th edn. Mosby, St Louis

Remedios L, Webb G 2005 Transforming practice through clinical education: professional supervision and mentoring. Elsevier, Sydney

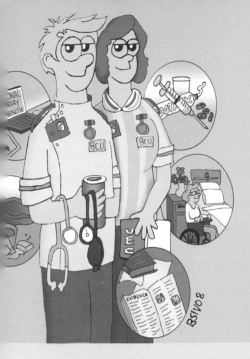

Chapter 6

Insights from clinical experts

Introduction

This chapter is a compilation of sections written by expert nurses. We are delighted to include the viewpoints and perspectives of people from a wide cross-section of nursing specialties as they introduce you to the particular learning opportunities and challenges inherent in diverse clinical areas. Of course, we haven't been able to cover every clinical specialty, but we hope that the selection included opens your eyes to the wonderful opportunities available to nursing students and to graduates.

6.1 Cancer care nursing

Kay Townsend

Lecturer and Locality Support of Learning in Practice,
University of Southampton,
Southampton, UK

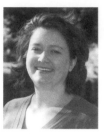

One in three people develop cancer during their lives and one in four people die from cancer. Although survival is improving, mortality from other diseases such as heart disease, stroke and infection is declining. Cancer became the most common cause of death in both sexes in the UK in 1995 (Office of National Statistics 2006). It is becoming increasingly likely that, whatever care setting you will work in once qualified, you will care for people who have or have had cancer.

John Diamond, the journalist, once said, 'Cancer is a word, not a sentence' (1999) about his own diagnosis of throat cancer. Too often, the reaction to hearing that someone has cancer is that their life is over. If you have been allocated a placement in an oncology setting, be it outpatients, primary, secondary or tertiary care, or a hospice, it is important that you know before you get there that your expectations and assumptions about cancer are likely to be inaccurate, either in part or extensively.

Assumptions are made because cancer is a little word that means too many things. Each one of the 200 cancers lumped together under the term 'cancer' behaves very differently, is treated differently, and has very different morbidity (the degree or severity of a disease) and mortality (death rate). Some cancers, for example testicular cancer, generally respond well to treatment, even when they are discovered after they have spread, whereas pancreatic cancer usually has a poor prognosis even when discovered early.

Another factor you will need to recognize is that the way in which people manage their reaction to being diagnosed with a cancer is also entirely individual, so the psychological care of this group of people is very diverse. As a result of this, you will look after people with a wide range of problems and there is a wide range of learning experiences available in this setting.

Challenges

This challenge is familiar to many nurses: how do we balance our personal feelings with our professional behaviour? Your personal experiences of cancer are just that, personal. Try not to let them overwhelm your placement. Of course, they will cloud how you empathize with others, but your role is to provide care for the patient with respect for their humanity and their need to form relationships with those around them. You need to be self-aware so that you do not bring sympathy and pity to work, but empathy and compassion. You will probably need to develop or refine your coping mechanism. To do this, I would recommend that you identify a peer, colleague or mentor to reflect with. Talking about your day or week in order to think about what happened, what you did well or felt you could have done better, and thinking about your reactions will be helpful in your growth as a professional in the care setting. This is what many nurses working in cancer care go through, and you are in an ideal position to find good role models.

Preparation for the placement

Research the following:

- The health page of the UK government website for national statistics provides a *general* picture of cancer across the country.
- Reflect upon people you have cared for in previous placements with cancer, and consider their illness trajectory and how this placement is similar or different.
- Choose one or two of the more common cancers to focus on (with more than 200 types of cancer, it is important to understand the principles rather than the particulars).

Learning opportunities

Whatever level of care, be it primary, secondary or tertiary, there are some common features of care in this client group. I would suggest that you consider:

- Social aspects of care – helping people to find out about ways to manage the financial consequences of being diagnosed with cancer. This may involve referral to social workers for benefits advice; help in identifying charitable sources of support; finding out about expert patient programmes; referral to a clinical nurse specialist.

- Communication – ask patients whom they think is a good nurse and then find out what it is that this nurse does differently to everyone else. What behaviours do you see them exhibiting that you could emulate?
- Understanding the patient journey – when you are spending time with a patient in a caring task, ask them if they would be happy to share what it's been like for them to be diagnosed with cancer.
- Visit the areas where patients are treated with chemotherapy and radiotherapy. Many areas have student information packs or patient information packs.
- Visit the outpatient clinics so that you can witness for yourself patients coming in for a check-up who have no recurrent disease. I hope that this will put the numbers of people diagnosed with cancer, and those that are cured or are surviving without problems, into perspective.

The survival of patients with in many types of cancer is improving. Some of these patients become critically unwell, either due to the cancer or to its treatment, and require care similar to that in high-dependency areas. Others will be nearer the end of life and require care that reflects the palliative care element. The section of this chapter written by Lucy Coggins explores palliative care in more detail.

References

Diamond J 1999 Because cowards get cancer too: a hypochondriac confronts his nemesis. Times Books, London

Office of National Statistics 2006 National statistics. Online. Available: http://www.statistics.gov.uk 12 Sept 2007

6.2 Community nursing

Sheila Jones

Practice Experience Manager,
Learning and Development Team,
St Leonard's Hospital, London, UK

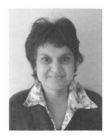

Community nursing is a specialized clinical practice area where nurses are involved in caring for clients in the community setting rather than the acute hospital environment. In the UK, community nurses are qualified general nurses with specialist training in their field of expertise, such as district nursing, health visiting and school nursing. They are autonomous practitioners who manage a caseload of clients in a specific geographical area and are usually based in community health centres, clinics or general practitioners' surgeries. Community nurses are also part of the primary healthcare team.

The main principles of community nurses work are:

- patient-centred care – using a holistic approach
- working within a skill mix team
- delivering quality and safe care to patients – adhering to standards and protocols
- collaborative networks – working with the multidisciplinary team and other agencies, such as social services, in order to have input in healthcare policy and decision-making
- using evidence-based practice – to provide high-quality, modern services and nursing care that is responsive to patient needs and the expectations of the 21st century.

Roles and responsibilities of community nurses

District nursing

The district nurse is a specialist practitioner with expert skills in the nursing care of the older person, the housebound, adults with complex health needs and those living in residential care settings. They are also knowledgeable in health promotion, and support patients in order to help them leave hospital sooner or to prevent them from being admitted to hospital.

Within their role, district nurses manage a team of nurses and ensure that care is appropriately planned, so that the team is involved in delivering nursing care to those who need it, while ensuring that other family members and/or carers receive the help, advice and support they require.

District nurses undertake holistic assessment, making referrals as appropriate by liaising with other healthcare professionals within the multidisciplinary team, to ensure that services are delivered efficiently and effectively to patients. Their workload varies tremendously, from simple dressings, monthly injections, to frequent home visits depending on client's needs. Some of the services provided by district nurses include:

- leg ulcer clinic
- participation in 'flu' vaccinations
- treatment room – dressings, removal of sutures.

Health visitors

The health visitor is a specialist practitioner who has experience and skills in child health, health promotion and education. Some of the services provided by health visitors include:

- breast-feeding support
- practical advice and support with infant feeding, sleeping and behavioural issues
- immunizations
- accident prevention
- health promotion and health reviews
- support for parents
- child protection
- sexual health advice
- offering support to any special needs that children have.

School nurses

The school nurse is a specialist practitioner with skills and experiences in the health of school-aged children as well as health promotion and health education; their role is to promote the well-being of school-aged children and the community as a whole. The following are some of the services that school nurses provide:

- contributing to school programmes – needs assessment of school health plans
- addressing health inequalities, such as obesity

- participating in parenting programmes
- sexual health advice
- child protection.

Preparation for a community nursing placement

Within this specialty placement, the practice experience manager/ facilitator will ensure that your journey is a smooth one and that your experience in the community is one of quality. You may also meet university link lecturers at either the induction, midpoint or evaluation of your placement period. Their role is to offer support and guidance to students and mentors.

To get the best out of your placement, you should have a good knowledge and understanding of the following core principles of nursing practice:

- professional codes of conduct
- ethics and accountability
- legal aspects of care, including consent for service and advocacy
- infection control
- documentation and confidentiality (client and staff)
- safety, security and manual handling.

Learning opportunities

It is expected that you will be working with a district nurse, health visitor, school nurse or registered community nurse who will be your named mentor throughout the placement period. Your mentor will provide you with understanding and insight into their roles and responsibilities, as well as the concept of community and primary care in the UK. You will also have opportunities to:

- spend time with other members of the skill mix team who will help you to develop your community experience
- explore one or many clinical specialty areas, such as tissue viability or practice nursing.

Learning outcomes

A placement within this specialty allows you to:

- benefit from discussion with practitioners, such as the community matrons, in relation to person-centred care and case management of patients with complex needs (that is, patients who have more than one long-term condition, such as having both a stroke and diabetes)

- recognize the shift in the balance of power when working with clients in their own home compared with that of the hospital setting
- become aware that a care plan is devised jointly with patients and carers, reflecting patient-centred care
- develop an awareness of partnership working and the importance of networking with other organizations, such social services, and the voluntary and independent sectors, such as hospices and private nursing homes.
- have the opportunity also to be involved in hands-on work and become increasingly aware of the public health role of community nurses in empowering their patients and clients to take responsibility for their own health
- develop insight into clients' journeys of health and illness
- begin to understand the involvement of carers, such as relatives, who look after a member of family (for example, frail older persons who wish to remain in their own home).

Challenges for students

It is important to remember that caring for clients in their own homes can present challenging learning situations as people live in a variety of settings, are from all walks of life, and have diverse backgrounds. This has implications for how nursing care is delivered and managed. Additionally, for some students, community nursing can seem less exciting and active than nursing in the hospital setting because you:

- may not be as involved as you would like to be because of the complexity and nature of the nursing care provided and the clinical expertise required
- may be confronted with the psychosocial risks and vulnerabilities that impact on some of the families with which community nurses work (this may include issues such as domestic violence)
- will be working with clients in their own environments, which involves accepting that the client has rights even when their perspectives and views differ from your own.

Community nursing as a career

Owing to changing patterns in health, illness and lifestyles, many people in the UK are requesting to be cared for in their own homes. The National Health Service needs appropriately qualified nurses who are 'fit for practice' and 'fit for purpose' to meet this demand in the community. This nursing specialty may well be a career that you will want to consider in the future, and for this reason it is important to prepare for and make the most of your placement in the community.

6.3 Critical care nursing

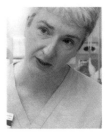

Maureen Coombs MBE

Consultant Nurse Critical Care, Cardiac Intensive Care Unit, Southampton University Hospitals Trust, and Senior Lecturer, University of Southampton, Southampton, UK

Have you ever wondered what goes on behind the doors of critical care? Is it really as portrayed on those well-known television programmes – all drama and crisis? What exactly do critical care nurses do? What I hope to do in this section is to dispel any myths or confusion you may have. My opening statement is that any nurse who chooses to work or undertake a placement in critical care has an amazing opportunity to support patients and families at a most vulnerable time in their lives. For me, in every sense, the critical care nurse works in an environment where *care is critical*.

What exactly is a critical care unit?

Critical care is a broad term encompassing intensive care or intensive therapy units (ICU/ITUs), and high dependency units (HDUs). The difference between these is how sick the patients are, and how much nursing and technical intervention is required. Generally each patient in ICU requires their own nurse to monitor and manage treatment interventions, and often requires ventilatory support (life support machines). In the HDU, patients will still be critically ill but have less severe disease processes, with perhaps only one body system failing (for example, cardiac or renal). Here you will often find one nurse caring for two patients. Within the wider healthcare system, specialty areas have evolved their own critical care areas, for example coronary care units (CCUs) and cardiothoracic ICUs. In addition, neurology, paediatrics and neonatal medicine specialties have there own critical care areas.

What goes on in critical care?

Within critical care, patients have potentially life-threatening illnesses or problems. These require an increased amount of nursing, medical, physiotherapy and pharmacy support. This results in a larger workforce than the wards. Most staff will have undergone further postregistration education to enable them to be safe and competent practitioners. Effective team working and collaboration of clinical teams should be a strong feature in critical care, ensuring that everyone contributes to and optimally manages patient care. As a result, you will be working alongside an entire army of potential educators!

You will notice that the essence of care in these units should be the same as in any other setting. Patient assessment and observation is used to direct and evaluate the treatment course, drugs and other interventions support normal physiology, and fundamental care promotes and sustains normal healthy tissue functioning. These are all important aspects of physical care. In addition to attending to care and support of the body, care and support of the mind and spirit are equally important. In critical care, the patient, family and loved ones come as one social unit needing support in some form.

In order to address all needs, the critical care nurse works in a structured and informed manner. On placement here, you will notice that each shift starts in a systematic way: a quick check of the patient, a full check of the safety kit and all the equipment and drugs that the patient is being supported by, and then a full head-to-toe assessment to inform planning for the day. Patient assessment is a detailed review of all body systems using physical assessment skills, laboratory and radiology test results; you will learn this systematic way of working. Patient observations are usually undertaken hourly, and are used to manage drug infusions, volume replacement and ventilator settings. Depending on the specialty of individual units, you will see nurses managing a range of machines and interventions, including cardiac monitors, ventilators, infusion pumps, under-water-seal chest drainage, haemofilters (renal therapy), intra-aortic balloon pumps, pacing and intracranial pressure monitoring.

Nursing is defined in a different way in critical care. Here, as part of the clinical team, the nurse works with patient and machine to support the patient's body and to work towards recovery. Patients who are ill and require ventilation will be sedated and therefore unable to perform even the simplest of functions – washing, cleaning their teeth, turning, even blinking at times. It is the nurse who must support these functions. In a good critical care placement, you will quickly realize that attending to these procedures is equally as important as the manipulation of pumps and infusions.

In essence, that which is provided in critical care supports the body systems until the patient recovers and their own systems are able to take over. This is what critical care provides: total patient support. Many patients get better and are discharged home, but, sadly, some patients do not survive. This is where a caring, supportive and understanding critical care nurse can ensure that the patient and family experience a respectful and peaceful death.

What are the learning opportunities?

In coming to critical care, the possibilities for learning are endless. Some key areas have been highlighted, including integrating knowledge bases, patient assessment, holistic care and team working. However, in critical care, you can learn so much more. Look back to the section above. In each sentence there are opportunities to think, question, practise, learn – and then start that cycle all over again! If that's not enough, how about these: the importance of asepsis in intravenous lines and drug administration; safe manual handling in unconscious, dependent patients; managing a safe working environment to pre-empt any emergency; prioritization and multi-tasking a workload; effective communication and decision making with medical and other healthcare staff; supporting distressed patients, families and staff. And that's just the tip of the iceberg.

How can you make the best of critical care?

Most students come to this placement in their second or third year, by which time they usually have a feel for where they want to work when they are qualified. You may come into critical care wanting to work in an acute or critical care unit, or may think that it is the last place in which you would want to work. Either way, think what you can learn from it. Ahead of your critical care placement, think what skills and knowledge you want to gain and what could be useful in future placements. If you are not going to work in an acute area, think, 'What skills are transferable?'. Think laterally and creatively, for there are many possibilities: systematic patient assessment, accurate documentation, breaking bad news, managing emergencies, effective team working. Think ahead; go with a plan of your learning needs. Trust me, there is nothing as demotivating for a mentor as an apathetic student. Take responsibility for your learning needs and help others to understand that you are there to learn. Now, think back over the last few sentences. It is not by chance that I have used the term 'think' several times. In this clinical placement, really think – if you do not, it may not be only the patient's lifeline that is at risk.

We understand that this is just one clinical area in which you will work, and that you will have many issues to contend with during your training, and many pressures to manage during your placements. However, if you have time, do some pre-reading (basic anatomy and physiology) and then let your further reading be led by what you learn. See whether there is a library on the unit, and use it. Ask your mentor what they think would be useful, and look for learning opportunities. If there is a re-intubation or admission, ask whether you can watch. Flag up your interest and you'll be amazed how people respond – it is noticed! If timely and appropriate, ask whether you can help, and remember your professional code of conduct. Never be afraid to say you need help or that you cannot, or should not, do something. Assert in a mature and professional way when you do not feel you are learning and developing. Critical care should be a supportive environment for patients and staff.

Critical care: the verdict

So, what's the conclusion? In my experience, students in critical care either love it or hate it. There are few who sit in the middle. You may have guessed from this personal account that I am as enthusiastic now for this challenging specialty as I was when I was a student nurse. I still have a passion about caring for critically ill patients and their families. I relish the opportunity to integrate anatomy, physiology, biochemistry, pharmacology, psychology and sociology science bases. I continue to be drawn to an area that requires close team working and, perhaps most importantly, working closely with the patient and their loved ones. I have been privileged and humbled to walk alongside many during critical illness and constantly learn about life, and death, from them. My hope is that you, too, gain and learn much from working in critical care, and that you offer respect to, and receive respect from, all those who share their experiences with you.

6.4 Emergency care nursing

Val Dimmock

Lecturer in Practice Education, Practice Theme Leader
City University, City Community and Health Sciences,
University College, London, UK

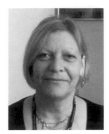

Emergency care in the UK focuses on trauma centres, accident and emergency departments, and minor injury units. You will gain emergency care experiences in one of these clinical placements. Your practice experience in emergency care will most likely take place when you are deemed to be a senior student. You will therefore have already developed skills and knowledge that you can build upon during this experience.

Any patient who becomes ill or injured 'unexpectedly' will be admitted through an emergency care unit for initial assessment, and then be transferred to an appropriate ward or department. To enable this type of care to be given effectively, staff are experienced in sound assessment techniques that will lead towards diagnosis and treatment. However, not all patients with whom you come into contact in these areas will be seriously ill or injured, and the skills that you will be refining relate to effective assessment of patients and making sound clinical judgements and decisions.

The nurse is often in the front line of assessing patients and requires technical knowledge, judgement and clinical decision-making skills in order to provide holistic care to patients and their families. Such support can be difficult and time-consuming during what is a traumatic time for both patients and families.

Trauma centres

Experiences arising from military conflicts have established the importance of minimizing the time from injury to definitive treatment and care. This concept has been extended to the management of civilian trauma and in the UK has led to the development of trauma centres. The distinguishing difference between these and accident and emergency departments is the *immediate availability* of specialized medical staff from all specialties, including surgeons, physicians, anaesthetists and nurses on a 24/7 basis. Accident and emergency departments may transfer their patients to specialized units if the specialty required is not available on site. Experiences in a regional trauma centre will develop your skills in providing leadership and holistic care for every aspect of injury.

Accident and emergency

Like any new experience, you will require time to settle into this environment before you can start to build on your existing nursing skills. This experience can introduce you to new challenges and practice, which will expand your existing knowledge of the bio-psychosocial, cultural and environmental aspects of health and illness. These environments offer students a vast number of learning opportunities, which can be overwhelming and may make it difficult for you to identify what you should be focusing on. All experiences have core principles, resulting in common learning opportunities. These include:

- accurate assessment skills for both minor and major conditions
- communicating with patients experiencing sudden or critical illness or injury
- caring and communicating with the patients' carers and significant others
- recognizing the deteriorating patient
- neurological observations and their significance
- accurate assessment of respiratory function
- use of a range of oxygen delivery devices, and an understanding of precautions and complications
- non-invasive and invasive ventilation
- suction
- tracheostomy care
- blood gases and their significance
- non-invasive and invasive monitoring techniques
- rhythm recognition
- ECG interpretation
- a working knowledge of central venous pressure measurement
- resuscitation and emergency equipment
- shock
- assessment of pain and the use of intravenous (IV) opiates
- nutrition and the critically ill patient
- fluid and electrolyte imbalance/balance

- acute renal failure
- organ donation
- transplantation
- pharmacology
- IV drug calculations
- immobility in the critically ill patient
- mouth care
- advocacy
- ethical dilemmas
- accountability
- death and dying
- working with the multidisciplinary team
- the expanded role of the nurse
- importance of accurate documentation.

You will probably not be exposed to all of the above learning opportunities, but awareness of what to look out for when you are caring for a patient requiring emergency care will give you a framework with which to organize your learning.

Emergency care requires a sound understanding of anatomy and pathophysiology, so you may need to refer to previous work in your course before commencing this experience. You may find it difficult to understand the complexities of assessment, intervention and the provision of treatment to these patients if you do not have a sound knowledge base of anatomy and physiology in the healthy person. Before commencing any emergency care experience it is important to think about the following:

- How long is it since I read about the anatomy and physiology of the respiratory, cardiac, gastrointestinal tract, neurological, musculoskeletal and renal systems?
- Do I understand how these systems work in health?
- What existing knowledge do I have on the subject of emergency care?
- How can I apply this knowledge to help me identify my learning needs?
- What is it that I would particularly like to gain from this experience?
- Am I particularly concerned about any area of knowledge and, if so, what can I do about it?
- Do I have clear learning outcomes for this clinical placement experience?

In the accident and emergency department a qualified nurse undertakes assessment of the patient. Up to 60% of patients attending accident and emergency departments are classified as non-urgent. A high proportion of these maybe assessed, diagnosed, treated and discharged by nursing staff without reference to a doctor.

Minor injury units

Emergency care nurses require specialist training and knowledge in order to deal not only with life and death situations but also with the minor injury side, which is developing into a specialty of its own. Minor injury units provide care for patients with less serious injuries, such as sprains, strains, cuts and grazes. Many people attend an accident and emergency department when they could be treated more easily, and probably more quickly, within a minor injury unit. In accident and emergency departments, staff give priority to serious and life-threatening conditions, so patients who attend with a minor injury will have to wait longer to be seen.

Minor injury units are run by emergency nurse practitioners, who have usually had previous accident and emergency experience. They treat a range of problems including:

- cuts and grazes
- sprains and strains
- broken bones
- bites and stings
- infected wounds
- minor head injuries
- eye problems (for example, minor infections or foreign bodies in the eye).

Patients with conditions that are usually not treated or given first aid by emergency nurse practitioners, and who are transferred to an accident and emergency department, include those with:

- chest pain
- respiratory problems
- abdominal pain
- gynaecological problems
- pregnancy-related problems
- drug overdose
- alcohol-related problems

- mental health problems
- conditions that would normally be treated by the general practitioner or hospital.

(NHS Direct 2007)

Summary

Remember that, to maximize the outcome for your patient, the principles of good emergency nursing are assessment, recognition of changes in their condition, clinical decision-making, intervention and treatment. This experience will be completely different to the experiences you have had working in the ward environments, and the pace of work varies dramatically – some days you may be run off your feet, and other days may be spent waiting for patients to attend.

You will already have many of the skills required for emergency care nursing, such as assessment, observational and communication skills. You will learn to build upon and enhance these skills during your experience. See below for one student's evaluation of the emergency care experience.

I was able to see the transition of the patient from accident and emergency department to the ward, to observe the baseline care and understand how it all worked. I now have a better understanding of drugs used in a cardiac arrest, BiPAP and CPAP. This placement has helped me realize that I can apply my nursing skills in various environments.

(Anonymous evaluation, third-year student nurse)

Reference

NHS Direct. Online Available: http://www.nhsdirect.nhs.uk Oct 2007

6.5 Forensic mental health nursing

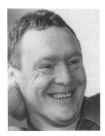

Barrie Green

*Forensic Nurse Consultant, Humber Centre for
Forensic Psychiatry, Humber Mental Health Teaching
NHS Trust, and Honorary Senior Lecturer,
University of Hull, Hull, UK*

Definition and overview of practice area

A student nurse placement in a forensic mental health environment
is an exciting, interesting and challenging experience. In the UK, the
range of service provision for mentally disordered offenders (MDOs)
includes high-, medium- and low-security hospitals, prison, court
liaison and community services, on a national, regional or local level.

'Forensic psychiatry' literally translates into meaning 'mental health
that relates to the law'. This is an interesting paradox, as in reality
all patients detained under the Mental Health Act 1983 are 'lawfully'
detained. In reality, the term generally indicates some measure of
patient involvement with the criminal justice system; however, not
all patients cared for by forensic teams are offenders, as the secure
services often provide care to physically challenging or dangerous
patients who cannot be managed in lower security hospitals.

The National Health Service provides the majority of services for
MDOs, but there is a growing number of private sector hospitals.
Most patients cared for by such services are adults of working age,
but there is a small number of child and adolescent medium-
security hospitals. There is also a growing number of people over
65 years of age who require a secure hospital placement. In addition, more recently a number of mental health in-reach services
have been developed in prisons that are often linked to local forensic teams. Increasingly, forensic services are part of an integrated
mental health and learning disability provision.

Multiprofessional, interagency functioning is well established in
most MDO services, of which the nursing contribution is central.
Traditional professional roles are therefore more flexible, with
cohesive teamwork being the focus of care.

Importance of the environment as a learning experience for nursing students

Since the widespread closure of the large institutions and the move towards community care, there has been a resultant reduction in opportunities for nursing students to develop their skills and knowledge relevant to inpatient environments. Since the early 1990s there has been a recognized need for the expansion and extension of secure and community mental health services. There are now several thousand secure hospital places in the UK, providing exposure to unique learning with regard to the skills required for this growing specialty. The focus is on treatment, risk management, recovery and rehabilitation within secure settings and within the community.

Students will develop their self-awareness and knowledge within a contemporary multidisciplinary environment, having exposure to situations of risk and danger, dual diagnosis, stigma and labelling, and serious and enduring mental illness. This will help to put forensic services into perspective, replacing the traditional stereotype of shadowy individuals, chains, dungeons and dark corridors, where the focus is on security and not treatment, and contrast it with a modern, dynamic, patient-centred model.

Learning opportunities

There are normally opportunities for students to experience several of the different service types during a placement with a forensic team. This can be either via formal placement within associated departments, or by participation in assessments, seminars or visits to other hospitals, courts, prisons or related patient placements. Many forensic services have robust interagency, clinical and academic links with services on a regional, national and international level; student exposure to these links is common.

The range of learning opportunities include:

- challenges to personal beliefs/stereotypes
- interpersonal aggression/violence
- research and evidence base
- multiprofessional working
- physical, relational and procedural security
- links between the criminal justice system and health services
- criminology and mental health

- offence analysis
- cognitive behavioural therapy – related to offending
- risk assessment and management
- dual diagnosis, including substance misuse/dependence
- personality disorder
- user and carer involvement.

Preparation for the placement

There are a number of negative perceptions that can colour a student nurse's selection of a secure or forensic placement. Therefore, these placements are normally facilitated in the later stages of training, usually as part of a specialist or elective placement. The chronology of this allows for the student to have developed a professional maturity and a broad understanding of the nature of mental disorder, and to have translated this into their practice. They should be confident in relation to multiprofessional teamwork and the unique role of nursing, and have an understanding of associated mental health legislation.

Students can be assured of one thing: that generally no two days are the same! They can expect to participate in very intense behavioural or psychiatric observations and assessments, highly technical integrated nursing care planning, and intricate treatment or rehabilitation interventions. Therefore, an open and mature approach is vital. Pre-placement visits, lectures and reading are important preparation.

Types of challenge

Most student nurses are excited at the prospect of a forensic placement, but some report initial trepidation. This can be anxiety provoking, particularly as they will be exposed to a range of unfamiliar situations. They will have quickly to orient themselves to the security protocols and legal procedures that are integral to functioning within secure environments or court-based situations. There is often an unfamiliar language used by experienced forensic professionals in everyday practice that is initially alien to newcomers. However, most forensic mental health services have comprehensive induction programmes that prepare new staff and students for practice.

A major dilemma for professionals, but more especially nurses, is a duality of role. The function of jailer and therapist must be integrated continually along a continuum of care and control. There are also challenges associated with either the nature of the offences or the stigma and isolation attached to the patients themselves. It is not unusual for human beings to experience shock, disgust or even a morbid curiosity at some of the background information and clinical interventions. To address these challenges, students must develop and practise unconditional positive regard, and be familiar with some psychotherapeutic mechanisms, including transference and countertransference. In addition, clinical supervision from an experienced mentor is essential.

Finally, and crucially, for all student nurses there must be an acceptance that this specialty is not for everyone. It should be accepted that such a placement is a time-limited exposure to a fascinating clinical and professional environment. Those who do not want to take this route as a career option will benefit from the exposure to the wide range of learning opportunities. However, for those who choose to return as a qualified nurse, the forensic mental health environment provides an excellent opportunity to develop their career in an expanding and diverse area of clinical practice.

6.6 Medical nursing

Maggie Maxfield

Practice Experience Facilitator,
Newham University Hospital NHS Trust,
London, UK

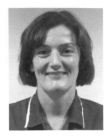

The acute care hospital comprises diverse care environments for inpatient services where secondary and tertiary levels of care are provided (Potter & Perry 2006). A medical ward is an area where inpatients are admitted under the care of physicians for the investigation or treatment of medical conditions not requiring surgical intervention. A medical placement can vary greatly, from an acute general ward in a district general hospital admitting patients with diverse medical conditions to a specialized medical ward in a large teaching hospital, which will have far more specific admission criteria, for example a renal unit or oncology. Both ends of the spectrum provide different but equally valid experiences. Some of the conditions you may meet while placed on a medical ward include:

* congestive cardiac failure
* left ventricular failure
* atrial fibrillation (arrhythmias)
* confusional states
* diabetes
* cerebrovascular accidents
* dehydration
* sickle cell
* HIV/AIDS and related disorders
* myocardial infarction
* unstable angina
* liver failure
* pancreatitis
* chronic obstructive airway disease
* asthma
* tuberculosis
* pneumonia
* leg ulcers
* anaemia
* gastrointestinal bleed

- enteral feeding
- pulmonary embolus
- deep vein thrombosis
- acute and chronic renal failure
- cancer care.

Medical patients are often admitted to the ward with a diverse range of conditions that can be confusing for you, making it difficult for you to relate the anatomy and pathophysiology of the patient and the subsequent care that is planned for that patient. You will often gain opportunities to practise the fundamental nursing skills with a wide range of patients and begin to understand the importance of viewing all patients as individuals. Remember that nursing is always patient centred.

The majority of nursing skills that you will perform for patient care can be undertaken in more than one way, requiring you to adjust your technique to suit the individual patient and yet still adhere to principles of practice (Nettina 2006). You may find that the complexity of the patient's condition makes it more difficult for you to interpret the observations of vital signs. For example, the baseline observations of a fit and healthy 20 year old will be different from those of an older adult with cardiac disease, but you need to know why, and to understand that what is normal for one patient may not be in the 'normal' textbook range.

You need to start being involved in administering medication to your individual patients as early as possible. Many of the medications that you come across will belong to common groups of drugs, for example antibiotics, analgesics and cardiac drugs. You need to start learning some of the common medications used, side-effects, cautions and routes. Administering medications can be quite nerve wracking at first, and you may find that your hands shake as you try to dispense medications into the receptacle in front of a qualified nurse. You may also feel that you are very slow and that you are holding up your mentor. Do not fear, you are not alone – everyone has been in your shoes. The sooner you do this, the easier it will be for you further on in your training. It is also important for you to familiarize yourself with the Nursing and Midwifery Council and Trust guidelines for the administration of medications (NMC 2002a).

The therapeutic relationship between nurse, patient, family and next of kin starts from the moment the patient walks through the door – how we greet, non-verbal cues, treating with respect, being polite, not over-reacting or taking offence to patient comments that are often made in times of stress. Sometimes it is important to explain to the patient why some things cannot be taken care of immediately, and to keep them informed about their condition. This has the overall aim of making patients feel safe and cared for, and developing a relationship of trust whereby the nurse acts as the patient's advocate. This therapeutic relationship lays the foundations for future emotional support, and possibly for dealing with difficult questions. The following tips can help:

- introducing yourself as a patient's named nurse for the day
- admitting lack of knowledge but willingness to find out
- undertaking a full assessment on admission
- spending time listening and answering questions.

Each medical ward will have its own culture and philosophy of care. You will gain far more from the placement if you seek to integrate and build relationships with the team and immerse yourself in the ward culture. You need to appreciate that your learning needs are important, but that the patients' needs will always come first. You need to take ownership of your own learning and make positive, proactive contributions to the team, which in turn will help you to meet your learning outcomes and result in a good working relationship between mentor and student. If you can demonstrate that you are able to participate actively within the ward setting, greater opportunities will arise. Some examples of the learning opportunities that you might access include:

- multidisciplinary forums – care planning meetings
- participating in ward rounds
- making referrals on behalf of patients to clinical nurse specialists, district nurses and discharge coordinators, to name but a few
- spending time with the clinical nurse specialists who link with the medical ward
- liaising with social workers, physiotherapists, occupational therapists, bed managers, site nurse practitioners, speech and language therapists, and dieticians.

It is important for you to identify and inform your mentor about what you need to know, and sometimes to remind them of what you already know and the level you are at in your training. Medical wards do not tend to have a routine, and you may be overwhelmed with information and find difficulty in identifying and extracting relevant information that needs to be passed on to other colleagues.

You need to maintain contact with the trained staff throughout the shift. The staff nurse may appear busy, but is still there to support and supervise you. It is important that you recognize the resources available to you on the ward, for example other students, healthcare assistants, clinical assistant practitioners, therapists and clinical nurse specialists. You should be contributing to shift handovers, and communicating verbally and in writing about your patients. The shift handover period is an ideal arena in which to develop your skills and confidence when handing over your patients, while providing an opportunity for clarification and teaching. As a senior student you will be expected to contribute to handover. As a junior student you should be encouraged to do this.

You should start to use the nursing process from the beginning of your training, reading care plans and writing about the care that you have given to your patients in the nursing notes. Correct and succinct documentation is very important in nursing, and you need to develop effective written skills. Nursing records need to be legible, grammatically correct and written in black ink, because they are documents that will be used by the multidisciplinary team and as legal evidence in the event of a complaint (NMC 2002b). All written entries in the nursing notes must be countersigned by a registered nurse, and this can provide an opportunity for you to gain feedback from your mentor/co-mentor.

You will finish each shift tired but satisfied that you have made a difference to someone who needed you. If you are prepared to become involved, to participate and to show your enthusiasm, you will feel the satisfaction that comes with being a valued team member.

Good luck and enjoy your nursing.

References

Nettina SM 2006 Lippincott manual of nursing practice, 8th edn. Lippincott Williams & Wilkins, Baltimore

Nursing and Midwifery Council 2002a Guidelines for administration of medicines. NMC, London

Nursing and Midwifery Council 2002b Guidelines for records and record keeping. NMC, London

Potter P A, Perry A G 2006 Fundamentals of nursing, 6th edn. Mosby, St Louis

6.7 Mental health nursing

Julie Attenborough

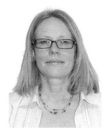

*Senior Lecturer in Mental Health Nursing, City
Community and Health Sciences, Incorporating St
Bartholomew School of Nursing and Midwifery,
London, UK*

Mental health nurses are the largest professional group working in
mental health services in the National Health Service, with nearly
40 000 staff (Department of Health 2004). Mental health nursing
provides a wide variety of experiences for students, with mental
health nurses found in many different specialist clinical settings,
including forensic mental health services, substance use, child and
adolescent mental health services (CAMHS), liaison mental health
services, sexual and martial services, eating disorders, self-harm
and elderly care.

Mental health nurses are required to work within the legislative
framework of the Mental Health Act 1983, under which people
can be detained for assessment and treatment. In the community,
people with mental health problems may be subject to aftercare
under the Act.

It is important to note that the majority of people with mental
health problems are treated in primary care. Common mental health
problems, such as anxiety and depression, are generally treated in
the primary care setting, depending on the severity of symptoms
and the effect on the person's life, whereas a minority of people
with serious mental health problems such as bipolar affective disorder and schizophrenia are managed by secondary mental health
services (Myles & Rushworth 2007). It is therefore important to be
aware that all nurses, not just those who chose to specialize in mental health nursing, will come into contact with people with mental
health problems.

'From values to action: The Chief Nursing Officer's review of
mental health nursing' (Department of Health 2006) recommends
some key steps to be taken to ensure best practice for the care and
treatment of people with mental health problems, based on promotion of social inclusion for service users and carers, use of the recovery model, and positive therapeutic relationships.

In relation to understanding the position of the service user and carer, students should have the opportunity to appreciate the service user's perspective of the experience of mental illness and of mental health services. One way of providing this is through meaningful input into nursing curricula by people who have been or who are users of mental health services and their carers, including those involve in the process of recruitment, training and curriculum planning, and assessment of mental health nurses (Simpson 2006).

The education of mental health nurses should stress the importance of maintaining therapeutic optimism, hope and belief in the concept of recovery (Perkins & Repper 2003). Belief in the possibility of recovery is crucial to mental health nursing, and it is important for students to understand the difference between 'recovery', 'rehabilitation' and 'cure'. By believing that a person who has mental health problems can live a purposeful life, mental health nurses contribute a great deal to the recovery process. It is vital that a range of options is available to a person with mental health problems, and that mental health nurses are aware of these and can help their clients to access and avail themselves of appropriate help.

Mental health care in the community

Much mental health care is provided in the community, and it is important to understand what services are available and whom they serve. The Mental Health Policy Implementation Guide (Department of Health 2001, 2002) is an extremely useful resource for understanding the work of these teams and how they relate to one another. Students would be advised to access this document before placement. Key ideas include:

- Community mental health teams (CMHTs) – give advice to other professionals about the management of mental health problems, whilst providing treatment and care for people in their own service.
- Assertive outreach teams (AOTs) – work with people who have severe and persistent mental disorders such as schizophrenia, and who have a high degree of impairment associated with their illness. The clients of AOTs tend to have high levels of admission to hospital or intensive home treatment, and complex problems and needs, such as forensic problems, use of substances in

addition to their mental health problem (dual diagnosis), or housing need. They also have difficulty in engaging with mental health services.

- Crisis resolution or home treatment teams – enable people with acute mental health problems to be treated in their own homes. They usually provide care and treatment 24 hours a day, 7 days a week.
- Early intervention teams – provide services to people in the early stages of developing psychotic illnesses, as this is linked to better outcomes for clients. The age range is 14–35 years.

Additionally, some areas have developed mental health in primary care teams, which provide a wide range of services and treatment options for people with mental health problems (Department of Health 1999).

Preparing for the placement

A wide range of materials is available via the internet for preparation purposes that students should access. In addition to knowledge about the range of mental health problems and the role of the mental health nurse, students should familiarize themselves with the structure of services. A basic understanding and knowledge of psychotropic drugs and physical interventions (such as electroconvulsive therapy) is also useful (Norman & Ryrie 2004).

Therapeutic use of self is very important in mental health nursing, and understanding the value of human relationships and communication skills cannot be overestimated. Students often say that they 'feel useless' and don't know what to say or how to behave when they are working with people with mental health problems. This is possibly due to fear of the unknown and unfamiliarity with the situation, and not really appreciating their most valuable asset – themselves. It is important that students are aware of and focus on developing the skills that they already have in order to become confident and effective in the mental health practice area (O'Carroll & Park 2007). There is also a need for structured clinical supervision to enable learning to be effective and safe; this will be provided through mentorship in mental health placements.

I hope that you enjoy your mental health placement, learn a lot about mental health, and also learn a lot about yourself.

References

Department of Health 1999 National service framework for mental health: modern standards and service models. DoH, London

Department of Health 2001 Mental health policy implementation guide. DoH, London

Department of Health 2002 Mental health policy implementation guide. DoH, London

Department of Health 2004 NHS hospital and community health service non-medical workforce census England 30 September 2003: detailed results. DoH, Leeds

Department of Health 2006 From values to action: The Chief Nursing Officer's review of mental health nursing. DoH, London

Myles P, Rushworth D (eds) 2007 A complete guide to primary care mental health. Robinson, London

Norman I, Ryrie I (eds) 2004 The art and science of mental health nursing. Open University Press, Maidenhead

O'Carroll M, Park A 2007 Essential mental health nursing skills. Elsevier Science, Edinburgh

Perkins R, Repper J 2003 Social inclusion and recovery. A model for mental health practice. Elsevier Science, Oxford

Simpson A 2006 Involving users and carers in the education of mental health nurses. Mental Health Practice 10(4):20–24

6.8 Midwifery

Jacqueline Gabriel-King

Lecturer in Practice (Midwifery),
City Community and Health Sciences,
London, UK

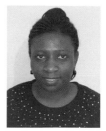

The practice environment

Working in the maternity setting and working beside midwives provides interesting and varied experiences. Midwives specialize in care during normal pregnancy and are also trained to provide care when things do not progress normally. As such, you will find midwives working in a variety of settings and in collaboration with the multidisciplinary team according to the needs of the individual woman.

Midwives provide holistic care to women from conception through the antenatal period, labour, birth and postnatal period up to 28 days after delivery. They play an important role in promoting health and detecting complications. When a pregnant woman is assessed as high risk, she is referred to the obstetrician and where appropriate collaborative care is carried out with a number of specialist midwives. For example, midwives specializing in conditions such as human immunodeficiency virus (HIV) infection, haemoglobinopathies, diabetes, and drug and substance abuse. Consultant midwives are also available, with remits in various areas such as public health and normal births. Their roles focus on improving women's services and addressing areas where there are poor outcomes such as infant mortality.

Midwifery care is geared towards the needs of women. Antenatal care is carried out in both the community and hospitals, with low-risk patients generally being seen in the community. Currently, most care in labour is carried out in hospital, in either high- or low-risk areas. The majority of hospitals have an allocated low-risk area for natural births. In these areas, midwives facilitate the use of natural methods. Examples include a pool for pain relief or water births, and use of balls and birthing chairs for alternative positions. Women with medical complications during pregnancy or those wanting interventions such as epidural anaesthesia for pain relief are cared for in an obstetric unit. Both areas usually function as a coherent unit, although some hospitals may staff the low-risk area separately. Regional neonatal intensive care units are available in larger maternity units. This may mean that in situations where serious complications occur, or when advanced care is required, women and their newborn babies may be transferred from a smaller hospital to a larger centre.

In the UK there is a major emphasis on women having choice in the services provided, in being well informed about the care they receive, and being actively involved in decisions that affect the care they receive. Various models of care exist such as midwife-run clinics, team midwifery, birth centre care and some community birthing services. A small number of women (1–3%) currently give birth at home. The aim of the government is to offer women even greater choice in the future. Midwives carry out safe and effective care, and they are all trained to carry out emergency measures for pregnant women while awaiting medical assistance.

The maternity environment offers a tremendous learning experience for student midwives, student nurses, medical students and others. It provides great insight into the high level of professional care required and is available to women who are experiencing a normal biological function. Further, it shows how expediently other resources and services can be implemented if complications arise, to ensure that risk factors are dealt with promptly.

Maternity care addresses the physical, psychosocial, cultural, spiritual and educational needs of the woman and her family. For example, parent education classes prepare couples for labour, birth, the postnatal period, care of the newborn baby and early parenting. Students will observe the supportive and educative role provided by midwives to support women throughout pregnancy, birth and the care of their newborn. Students also need to be mindful that the outcome of pregnancy is not always a happy one for all women. Stillbirth and neonatal death are a reality for some, in spite of the expert services available.

Bereavement services offering counselling and support are also part of the midwife's remit.

After delivery, early discharge of well women and their babies is encouraged. Upon discharge from hospital, mothers are provided with a discharge package with information on local community contact numbers and support groups to assist and support them with newborn and infant care. Community midwives visit women and babies in their homes to continue care. This includes infant screening, breast-feeding support and early detection of problems such as postnatal depression. The introduction of midwives at children's centres in some areas offers healthy postnatal women the option of bringing their babies to clinics instead of waiting to be seen by the midwife at home. When the community midwife discharges the mother and baby from care, the health visitor and general practitioner continue to contribute to the maintenance of their health.

Learning opportunities

Antenatal

Antenatally, the health and well-being of the woman and the developing fetus is paramount, with emphasis on nutrition and healthy lifestyle. Learning opportunities include:

- observing and participating in antenatal booking of pregnant women, including screening and risk assessment
- providing care during normal pregnancy, including monitoring fetal well-being with non-invasive methods such as Pinnards and Sonicards
- observing the service provided for pregnant women with medical complications such as pregnancy-induced hypertension, gestational diabetes, HIV and various infections
- understanding how parentcraft classes assist couples in preparing a birth plan ready for the labour.

Birth

During pregnancy the focus of most couples is on the impending labour. The care and attention of a new baby becomes the predominant thought after the birth. During labour, students will learn of the close monitoring necessary to prevent or detect any deviations from the norm. An understanding of the physiology of labour becomes essential. The role of the midwife in providing physical and psychological support to the woman and her support person becomes evident.

Pain in labour has a functional role. Strong painful contractions are needed to move the fetus through the birth canal. Therefore, physiological pain is an expectation of labour. Women's ability to tolerate pain varies, and the midwife supports them in the choice of various options for pain relief.

Non-pharmacological pain relief such as massage, various positions, warm showers and breathing techniques are offered to women. Pharmacological methods include pethidine, diamorphine and epidurals.

Physical assessment of the progress of labour and fetal monitoring are carried out before administering these drugs. Most medications used cross the placenta and affect the fetus; the midwife therefore takes timing into consideration when administrating any drug in order to reduce the risk of respiratory depression at birth. Further, the mother is preloaded with an intravenous infusion to prevent hypotension after the administration of epidural analgesia.

The second stage of labour requires a lot of maternal effort. It is at this time that the student will see a range of different cases. Experiences range from observing maternal behaviours in the natural setting to obstetric interventions in the form of ventouse delivery, forceps delivery or caesarean section. Midwives and obstetric staff all participate in regular updates in emergency obstetric procedures. This is to ensure quick team effort in emergencies such as postpartum haemorrhage, shoulder dystocia or breech delivery. Soon after normal birth, midwives deliver and inspect the placenta and membranes to ensure that they are complete. They examine the perineum, suture any episiotomy or lacerations, and ensure that bleeding is controlled. Further observations and detailed documentation of the entire birthing process, the cord bloods and the identification of the newborn, initiation of breast-feeding and handover completes the process.

Postnatal

The first 24 hours after birth is a crucial time for mother and baby. Monitoring of vital signs, physical assessment for involution of the uterus, lactation advice and support of breast-feeding will be just some of the care given to the mother. It is an adaptation period for baby and requires physical assessment, observation and documentation of vital signs, feeding behaviour and excretory functions.

The opportunity to debrief the parents about the birth allows for questions to be addressed and explanations to be given. This plays an important part in promoting psychological well-being. Midwives also encourage women to develop an early and long-lasting relationship with their babies by promoting rooming-in, education and support. Students can observe the behaviours and rituals practised by some mothers that are based on cultural traditions; for example, some Asian women delay breast-feeding.

Preparing for the placement

Students should prepare for the placement by reading about maternity care and make some notes on the following:

- the purpose of antenatal care
- the stages of labour
- the differences between a natural birth and an operative delivery
- the purpose of postnatal care
- rationales for women having a hospital stay after birth
- the need for some specialist services.

Listening to birth experiences of family and friends will help you to gain insight into what can be expected.

Staying focused

Use your portfolio of activities to assist you in planning relevant learning objectives on a daily basis. Review the objectives mid-placement with your mentor or lecturer in practice to ensure that you are meeting the essential clinical experience of the placement.

Be aware that maternity services promote women participating in their own care. When on placement, observe how they do this and learn from them how they put together a plan for pregnancy and birth.

Students may experience a feeling of inadequacy and be overwhelmed by the clinical environment. This is a common feeling among students; be guided by your link lecturer, personal tutor and mentor. Your allocated midwife will tell you what he or she is doing and why, and will have most of the answers to your questions. Reflect on one day at a time in preparation for the next day, be realistic, and don't expect too much of yourself. Identify and explore challenges during each placement.

Challenges for the student

Some clinical areas, such as the antenatal clinic and postnatal ward, are frequently very busy; this may be rather daunting initially. Don't despair; the team leader is very proficient in ensuring that women's needs are being met. Your mentor will assist you in adjusting to this new environment. Just prepare yourself to expect some degree of chaos. The postnatal ward, for example, has three main activities: women wanting physical care and assistance, others preparing for discharge, and admission of women and babies from the delivery suite.

Labour and birth

Your first experience of labouring women may be challenging: you may react to the physical appearance of the woman in labour, nudity and even the noises she may make. Expect to be on a steep learning curve and reflect on what you have read about the physical, psychosocial, spiritual and cultural aspects of labour. One can never be adequately prepared for witnessing birth, as it is a very emotional journey for some.

Complications

Obstetric and medical problems can occur in pregnancy, labour, birth and the postnatal period. An awareness of some of the complex situations that require medical intervention will confirm the importance of monitoring and early intervention to ensure good outcomes. Experience in the clinical area will challenge your need to learn more about assessment, diagnosis and management in pregnancy.

Cultural sensitivity

Being culturally sensitive is as important as being competent in delivering physical care. Women and their family support members may require extra care based on needs. Depending on the area of your placement, you will encounter women from various cultural and religious backgrounds. Staff such as the health advocate will support those speaking different languages. You will also learn of the different diet and religious needs of various groups.

Loss and grief

Loss, in broad terms, may mean a woman's lost opportunity for something she had planned to gain from her pregnancy and birth or postnatal experience. For example, she may have planned to labour without pharmacological medications but succumbed to using an epidural after prolonged labour. She may have wanted a natural birth but had to have an operative delivery because of fetal complications, or perhaps she chose formula to feed her baby because of overwhelming difficulties with breast-feeding. The sense of loss that women feel can be helped by acknowledging their feelings and providing an opportunity for debriefing. The loss of a baby or mother in maternity care is rare, but is felt intensely by family and attending staff.

Conclusion

A midwifery placement is challenging and rewarding. To experience the process is amazing. It will enhance your personal and professional development, and enable you to reflect on natural and complex situations as you develop as a nurse, midwife or doctor.

Further reading

Department of Health 2004 Maternity services: national service framework for children, young people and maternity services. DoH, London
Department of Health 2007 Making it better: for mother and baby. DoH, London
Department of Health website: http://www.dh.gov.uk
Henderson C, Macdonald S 2004 Mayes' midwifery: a textbook for midwives, 13th edn. Baillière Tindall, London
Royal College of Midwives 2007 Home births. Joint Statement No. 2. Royal College of Obstetricians and Gynaecologists/Royal College of Midwives, London. Online. Available: http://www.rcm.org.uk/info/docs/Home%20Births_Joint%20Statement.pdf 25 Feb 2008
Royal College of Midwives website: http://www.rcm.org.uk
Stables D, Rankin J 2005 Physiology in childbearing with anatomy and related biosciences, 2nd edn. Elsevier, Edinburgh

6.9 Older person nursing

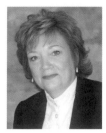

Hazel Heath

Independent Consultant on Nursing and Older People,
Honorary Senior Research Fellow at City University
London, London, UK, and Consultant Editor to the
Journal of Dementia Care

Working with older people

Older people can be the most fascinating, rewarding and enjoyable individuals to nurse. With decades of accumulated experience, they offer to nurses a richness of perspectives and their unique individual wisdom.

There is a tendency in contemporary Western society to describe older people as 'the elderly', as if all these individuals have common characteristics and common needs. In reality, older adults are highly diverse – for example, the last of the First World War veterans who in 2007 celebrated his 111th birthday, early pioneers of Rock 'n' Roll now in their seventies and eighties, or people who have lived for most of their lives on the other side of the world and who are now growing old in the UK.

Although older people have lived different lives to younger people, it is worth remembering that we are all ageing as, along life's journey, we build our unique biographies. Fundamentally, whether young or old, healthy or sick, we all experience human relationships, joys and frustrations, fond memories and hopes for the future.

Older people are the major client group in most health and social care services, and it is therefore essential that all nurses understand how to care for them. Working with older people can offer rich learning experiences for nursing students, and hopefully many will want to develop specialist expertise in gerontological nursing.

This section outlines key issues, challenges and potentials in the hope of enthusing nursing students to want to learn more about the opportunities and professional fulfilment that working with older people can offer.

Maximizing learning opportunities

The interrelationship between individuals, lifestyles, normal ageing and health is complex, and students need to learn how to unpick these complexities in order to offer effective care (Heath & Watson 2005).

Ageing and health/illness: We age individually: our physiological systems age in different ways and at different rates. Genetics and lifestyles influence how we age and the health or illness we experience. This may be distinct between generations; for example, in older people's formative years, smoking, radiation and asbestos were not recognized as major causes of lung cancer.

Distinct disease patterns in later life: Some illnesses, such as dementia, occur mainly in later life, although this disease sometimes affects younger people and also those with Down syndrome.

Multiple pathology: The older we become, the more diseases we tend to experience. It is not uncommon for people in their eighties and nineties to have four or more medical diagnoses.

Altered presentation of illness: Primarily due to the physiological effects of ageing, symptoms can manifest differently in older people. Common 'altered presentations' of illness are physical instability, mental instability, immobility or incontinence ('the four Is'), but symptoms may be subtle. Delirium (acute confusion) can be the first sign of life-threatening illness and must be investigated urgently (Schofield 2007).

The 'domino' effect: Because ageing reduces the effectiveness of our adaptive mechanisms, one problem tends to exacerbate another, thus starting a 'domino effect' leading to decline, health or social breakdown, and even death.

'Polypharmacy': To treat multiple pathology, multiple drugs are often prescribed but these can interact and result in adverse drug reactions.

Communication: Learning to communicate with people who have difficulty with hearing or sight, or who have dementia or stroke, requires sensitivity and skill.

Mental capacity: New legislation around the UK places increased emphasis on assessing a person's capacity to make decisions and to give informed consent.

Carers and families: Balancing the needs and wishes of carers or families with those of the older person requires professional judgement and skill.

Maintaining networks and social activities: In order to help older people maintain their daily life activities, friendships or income, nurses need to know how to engage with other agencies such as social services, housing or transport.

Multiprofessional, multidisciplinary and multiagency working: For care to be effective, older people require coordinated responses from a range of health and social services and specialist professionals. Experiencing the realities of interdisciplinary working can be immensely valuable for nursing students.

Addressing challenges

Working in services for older adults can be challenging, but it is important to recognize that many of the challenges do not originate from older people themselves. Rather, they highlight inaccurate perceptions and the need for a greater understanding of how to work most effectively with older individuals.

Remaining positive: Ageism and negative stereotypes depict ageing as an inevitable physical decline or 'losing one's marbles', and lead to low expectations in terms of the potential to improve older people's health or functioning. If older people do not receive appropriate treatment or care, this can become a self-fulfilling prophecy.

Crossing generational barriers: Nurses can be four generations younger than the patients they work with, and achieving understanding is not always easy. Young students may find it difficult to empathize with someone who has lived through experiences they cannot contemplate, such as world war, genocide or famine. Conversely, older people have described how their values and priorities can seem out of touch in a technological age.

Coping with vulnerability, disability or death: If you have never experienced profound disability, dying or death, working in units where these are the everyday realities, and particularly giving intimate and supportive care, can be difficult.

Coping with challenging situations: People who are ill or vulnerable, and particularly those with mental health needs, can behave in ways that challenge those who try to care for them.

Recognizing the expertise needed to nurse older people effectively: The high levels of expertise needed to nurse older people are not always recognized. Medicine and nursing with older people was historically seen as 'basic' and not accorded high status.

Promoting best practice

Learning how to care for older people and developing specialist expertise in gerontological nursing are vital both now and in the future.

Nursing has a distinct contribution to make to older people in terms of:

the use of clinical judgement in the provision of care to enable people to improve, maintain, or recover health, to cope with health problems, and to achieve the best possible quality of life, whatever their disease or disability, until death

Royal College of Nursing (2003, p 1)

Building on this, gerontological nursing has been defined as: 'a person-centred approach to promoting healthy ageing and the achievement of wellbeing, enabling the person and their carers to adapt to health and life changes and to face ongoing health challenges' (Kelly et al 2005, pp 14–15).

The clinical expertise of nurses can be critical in older people's care. Good nursing assessment can anticipate and identify health problems. Good nursing intervention can prevent complications and delay the development of disability. Good nurses offer comfort and peace of mind towards the end of life (Heath 2006).

When challenges arise, it is important to identify the reasons for these. The more we understand, the more constructively we can address the causes. Sometimes further knowledge can help. For example, contrary to perceptions of ageing as decline, research demonstrates that exercise can improve muscle strength and that healthy lifestyles can considerably improve health even into very old age.

Good role models can identify helpful approaches or resources. Effective, ongoing support is essential, and students should seek help from mentors with expertise in nursing older people and a positive attitude to this.

Perhaps most importantly, nursing students should spend time with older people, listening to their views and stories. If nurses approach older people as individuals, each within the context of a unique biography encompassing perceptions of past, present and future, we are better placed to help them. Creative, proactive and dynamic nursing that addresses the priorities of older individuals can contribute significantly to their health, well-being and quality of life.

References

Heath H 2006 No substitute for nurses. Nursing Standard 21(10):19–21

Heath H, Watson R 2005 Older people: assessment for health and social care. Age Concern, London

Kelly T B, Tolson D, Schofield I, Booth J 2005 Describing gerontological nursing: an academic exercise or prerequisite for progress? Journal of Clinical Nursing 14(suppl 1):13–23

Royal College of Nursing 2003 Defining nursing. RCN, London

Schofield I 2007 Delirium. In: Neno R, Aveyard B, Heath H (eds) Older people and mental health nursing: a handbook of care. Blackwell, Oxford, p 168–181

Resources

Websites: Older people's organizations such as Age Concern, Help the Aged, Alzheimer's Society

Nursing organizations with learning resources for students: Royal College of Nursing

Journals: International Journal of Older People Nursing (Blackwell Publishing), Nursing Older People (RCN Publishing), Journal of Dementia Care (Hawker Publishing)

Comprehensive textbooks, such as:

Heath H, Schofield I 1999 Healthy ageing: nursing older people, Mosby, London

Redfern S J, Ross F M 2006 Nursing older people. Churchill Livingstone Elsevier, Edinburgh

6.10 Paediatric nursing

Jeremy Jolley

Senior Lecturer in Paediatric Nursing,
Faculty of Health and Social Care,
University of Hull, Hull, UK

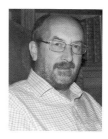

Children's nursing is one of the most rewarding areas of nursing. We all understand that children are precious to their parents and to others who know them. In fact, there exists no stronger human emotion than the love that parents feel for their children and the love that children have for their family. When a child becomes ill or is injured, the family is at its most helpless. It follows that working with sick children and their families is a great privilege – and not every nurse is able to meet the challenge. Being a children's nurse is to be with the child and family at one of the most important times in their lives; it is to share, with both the child and the family, their anxiety, fear, pain and joy. In no other field of nursing is it so necessary to 'get inside the head' of the patient. This is important because children may not be able to communicate verbally, either because they are too young to do so effectively, because they are ill, or simply because they choose not to share their feelings with another person.

Children's nursing is not a field of nursing where the nurse can elect to be detached from the emotional world being played out around them. So, to be a children's nurse is to feel the child and family's pain. However, it is also one of the most fulfilling and pleasurable areas in which a nurse can work. Children are amazing human beings, and their sense of fun and their sheer propensity for happiness rubs off on those around them.

It is impossible to nurse the child without also nursing the family. On any typical children's ward, there will be parents everywhere, and grandparents and brothers and sisters, all reflecting the value of the sick child's life. Children's nurses must want to work with the family as much as they want to work with the child. The typical children's ward may be a clean place, but it is never tidy. Play is a way we have of communicating with children and they with us. Play is rarely a 'tidy' event and it follows that a tidy ward is hardly suitable for children. In the same way, children's nurses need to be flexible and imaginative. Procedures often designed for adult patients may be inappropriate or need adapting to the needs of the child. In children's nursing, the rulebook is rewritten with every child admitted to our care.

Children tend to stay in hospital only during the acute stage of the illness or treatment. Many children are cared for at home, even those receiving quite technical care. Here, the nurse is able to provide advice and direct technical care that may be too complex for the parents to manage themselves. It is often the case, however, that the family can feel very much on their own at home. In this situation, the community children's nurse can be useful in assessing the child and reassuring the family that everything is as it should be. It has long been recognized that the hospital environment is not the best place for a child. Despite everyone's best efforts, the hospital can be frightening and it can never provide the proper environment within which a child can grow up normally. By providing expert care to the child at home, the community children's nurse makes it possible for the child to be discharged from hospital much earlier than would otherwise be the case.

Your paediatric allocation will provide a rich learning experience. You will want to find out why these children have been admitted to hospital. However, it is just as important to get to know the child and family, and to spend time with them. Try to think what it must feel like to be in hospital as a child, how vulnerable and powerless you would feel. Try to think about what you would make of all the equipment and machinery, and how you would feel if your parents were not there with you. It is these and many other fears that the nurse has to anticipate. The nurse must try to make the physical and interpersonal environment one in which the child can feel comfortable and 'at home'. However, children's nurses do more than this: they try to make the child's time in hospital an enjoyable one.

In general hospitals you will find that the children's ward takes children from almost every medical and surgical specialty. There may be children with orthopaedic injuries in the same ward as babies with heart problems and adolescents with mental health problems. The children's hospitals provide more specialist care, and here you will find that children's nursing is at least as technical, modern and complex as any other area of nursing.

There are many texts for students anticipating their first paediatric placement (e.g. Glasper & Richardson 2005). You will also find it useful to review your understanding of the stages of child development (see Sheridan et al 1997). In addition, you should at least be aware of the vital signs of children, such as pulse rate and blood pressure, at different ages and be familiar with the normal range of height and weight of children (see Paxton et al 2005). It is also useful to understand basic fluid balance, and you should know how to calculate a drug dosage (see Gatford & Phillips 2006). Children are not small adults: they are different psychologically, medically and in just about every other conceivable dimension (Chamley et al 2005).

If children's nursing is for you, you will know it by the end of your first allocation. You will have learned more than you thought it was possible to learn. You will have 'grown' inside because of what you have seen and experienced. Some of these experiences will have been difficult for you, but you will also have had fun – lots of fun. Importantly, you will have begun to learn what it is that is so special about children's nursing.

References

Chamley C, Carson P, Randall D, Sandwell M 2005 Developmental anatomy and physiology of children. Elsevier, London

Gatford J, Phillips N 2006 Nursing calculations, 7th edn. Churchill Livingstone, London

Glasper A, Richardson J 2005 A textbook of children's and young people's nursing. Churchill Livingstone, Edinburgh

Paxton G, Munro J, Wilkinson D 2005 Paediatric handbook. Blackwell Science, Oxford

Sheridan M, Frost M, Sharma A 1997 From birth to five years: children's developmental progress. Routledge, Oxford

6.11 Palliative care

Lucy Coggins

Lecturer Practitioner in Palliative Care,
University of Southampton and Oakhaven Hospice
Trust, Lymington, UK

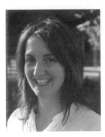

In my experience, palliative care is a specialty that elicits different responses from different people. At one end of the spectrum some can enthuse passion and commitment when working with people and families facing the end of life, while at the other the response can take the shape of 'Oh, I don't think I could do that ... isn't it depressing?'. Whatever your initial response, a placement in palliative care will offer you wonderfully diverse learning opportunities.

Palliative care can be defined as 'an approach that improves the quality of life of patients and families facing the problems associated with life-threatening illness, through the prevention and relief of suffering by means of early identification and impeccable assessment and treatment of pain and other problems, physical, psychosocial and spiritual' (Sepulveda et al 2002). Over several decades the provision of palliative care services has evolved significantly. Many years ago palliative care was associated with only the hospice setting, where care at the very end of life was provided for those with cancer. In today's society palliative care services can be found in the community, acute hospital settings, care homes and the hospice environment. The push to introduce such care earlier on in the patient disease trajectory is also evident, moving away from care only at the very end of life. The inclusion of those with non-malignant disease is also an important development within this field, extending the benefits of such care to many more with incurable illness.

Learning opportunities

The following is by no means an exhaustive outline of learning opportunities, but may be considered some of the more overarching themes evident.

A palliative care placement will give you the opportunity to gain insight into holistic assessment, planning, implementation and evaluation of care for patients and families at this difficult time in their lives. Two patients with very similar diseases may have two completely different experiences of living with dying and death. The holistic approach to care can ensure that individualized care is provided in an attempt to support and improve quality of life and death in ways that are most appropriate to each patient and family.

In order to achieve the above, multidisciplinary team working is essential. Doctors, nurses, physiotherapists, occupational therapists, religious or spiritual ministers, complementary therapists, counsellors and pharmacists often participate in the complex discussions and decision-making involved within palliative care. A placement within this specialty will not only provide opportunities for you to observe and become involved in such decision-making and discussion, but will also draw on the knowledge and skills of the multiple disciplines involved. Having access to 'many brains to pick' can provide greater insight and understanding of the diseases seen within palliative care, the medications and treatments often used in symptom control, and the different perceptions and opinions that can arise around different aspects of care.

Excellent communication skills are paramount in palliative care and, again, a placement in this field may help you develop such skills. Whether observing others as they participate in difficult conversations with patients and families around end-of-life decision-making, enhancing your assessment skills through good communication, or simply gaining reassurance that even those with years of experience still struggle at times with 'the right thing to say', these experiences will improve your confidence and communications skills. These skills are transferable to any area of nursing practice – let's face it, you would be hard pushed to find a nurse who has never had to deal with an emotional or distressed patient, or angry relative, or been asked what can be deemed a 'difficult question'.

Preparation for placement

Every individual will have their own perceptions about death and dying. An important element of preparation will be to reflect on your own personal experiences and beliefs, and how these may affect your responses, attitude and ultimately the care you provide. Being aware of your thoughts and feelings before starting the placement will help if you are faced with challenging and emotional situations. It may help you articulate to colleagues and mentors if you have specific concerns, or explain why you feel the way you do. Reflecting in this way will help you to see how you may develop throughout the placement and how your thoughts and feelings may alter with knowledge, experience and deepening insights.

Challenges

As with any placement, a diverse range of challenges may present themselves and to predict them all would be impossible. However, within the specialty of palliative care, perhaps the most pertinent is the emotional challenges that you may experience. Exposure to suffering, at times unrelieved symptoms and potentially multiple losses is undoubtedly difficult. Some nurses have personal coping mechanisms that help; others are still in the process of discovering or developing these. The staff you work with will be experienced and are themselves human beings affected by such events. They are there to help, support and guide you if needed. Who better to understand the emotions and challenges involved in palliative care than those who you will be working with? Being open and receptive to experiences, and seeking support and advice from colleagues and mentors, are essential strategies for gaining the most from your placement.

Finally, remember that palliative care can be, and often is, surrounded by appropriate laughter. So go to your placement, laugh, cry, but most of all enjoy and learn!

References

Sepulveda C, Marlin A, Yoshida T, Ullrich A 2002 Palliative care: the World Health Organization's global perspective. Journal of Pain and Symptom Management 24(2):91–96

6.12 Perioperative care during anaesthesia and surgery

Paul Wicker

Head of Operating Department Practice,
Edge Hill University,
Liverpool, UK

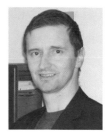

Introduction

Registered nurses and registered operating department practitioners (ODPs) working in the operating department provide perioperative care to patients before, during and after anaesthesia or surgery. Patients may need perioperative care in many other environments too, including, for example, general practice surgeries, X-ray departments, accident and emergency departments and intensive care.

Nursing students in the UK usually experience the perioperative environment as a short placement lasting for perhaps 6–10 weeks, or accompanying individual patients through the various stages of their anaesthesia or surgery. Your requirements for learning are therefore likely to be different to those of student ODPs, whose main learning resides in perioperative care. This section describes the learning opportunities and challenges that you will meet when spending a short time in perioperative care as part of a larger programme of study.

Pre-registration nursing students working in perioperative care have opportunities to experience a wide range of acute episodes involving patients and to take part in many different clinical procedures.

Learning opportunities

Many operating departments offer students excellent orientation and induction packages to help them to become integrated into the culture of the perioperative environment.

You will enter the perioperative environment with the need to learn the competencies required for your registration. These are in the domains of professional/ethical practice, care delivery, care management and personal/professional development.

Learning opportunities in professional/ethical practice

Examples:

- You will need to assess your own level of competence while practising the roles of circulating nurse, scrub nurse and recovery nurse, in order to understand the boundaries to those roles.
- You may face situations where confidentiality is paramount, such as during sensitive procedures, when the patient is semi-conscious, or when giving information to family, friends or colleagues.
- You will learn about the importance of documentation for delivering effective patient care, for example recording swab checks, checking consent forms and completing operating department records.
- You will test your own accountability by understanding the accountability required when checking instruments before procedures, employing particular techniques such as cricoid pressure, and managing your own workload and responsibilities within the surgical team.
- You will face ethical and professional situations and dilemmas that need to be resolved, for example consent in under 16 year olds, giving information to parents, and working with patients from varied cultural backgrounds.

Learning opportunities in care delivery

Examples:

- You will learn how to provide an ideal environment for care, taking into account factors such as appropriate clothing, equipment, the environment and asepsis.
- You will learn how to provide evidence-based individualized care by appraising the potentially rapidly changing patient condition, applying knowledge of wound management, positioning patients safely, managing pain relief, and understanding the significance of normal and altered human anatomy and physiology.
- You will apply understanding and knowledge of pharmacology in perioperative care, for example anaesthetics, sedatives, tranquillizers, muscle relaxants and antibiotics.
- You will be exposed to a wide variety of medical devices that support the care of patients, for example ECG machines, anaesthetic machines, diathermy, suction, Dopplers, video stacks for minimally invasive surgery and endoscopic equipment. You will also develop an understanding of the need for good training

techniques, support from company representatives, and procedures for the introduction and use of medical equipment.

- You will be exposed to the main roles in the operating department of anaesthetic, scrub and circulating practitioners.
- You will gain an understanding of effective communication skills
and methods, for example notifying the surgical team of changes
to the operating list, discussing procedures with patients before
surgery, listening to patients' concerns about surgery, telling
surgical teams of the availability of instruments or equipment,
and completing documents, such as specimen forms, telephone
messages and operating book records, accurately.

Care management

- You will learn how risk assessment can help to increase patient
and staff safety, for example risk assessment of the environment
(e.g. height of shelves, lifting trays, maintaining temperature)
and the use of dangerous substances (e.g. glutaraldehyde and vol-
atile anaesthetic agents).
- You will gain opportunities to work with a diverse team of professionals, including consultant surgeons and anaesthetists, junior
doctors, qualified nurses and ODPs, radiographers and medical
scientists.
- You will learn how to delegate effectively and the responsibilities
assumed and transferred when one practitioner delegates work to
another.
- You will learn how to record information effectively using various
methods, for example operating theatre electronic records,
patient documentation, operating lists, specimen forms, theatre
checklists and patient handover information.

Personal/professional development

For example:

- Working under supervision, you will face new situations that will
require you to gain knowledge or learn techniques in advance.
These include taking part in surgical and anaesthetic procedures
such as intubation, extubation, insertion of central lines, urinary
catheterization, and working as scrub nurse for procedures such
as release of carpal tunnel, appendicectomy, fracture reduction
and fixation, and hysterectomy.

- You will develop an understanding of the value of 'debriefing' following critical incidents or important events, such as cardiac arrest, respiratory obstruction, sudden hypotension, onset of acute pain, haemorrhage or other sudden changes in the patient's condition.
- You will be able to identify your own learning needs through reflection on perioperative events. By reflecting on the care given to patients during surgery you may identify areas in which you could improve.
- You may be able to contribute to developing learning resources in the area, for example through writing a patient information leaflet, undertaking a literature search about a procedure or writing about your experiences in the theatre area.

Preparing for the placement

The perioperative environment is an exciting and challenging area, offering opportunities to develop a wide range of skills, knowledge and experience. It is essential that you prepare for this experience so that you gain the most benefit.

Self-directed learning

A major resource for information about the perioperative environment is available from the Association for Perioperative Practice (AFPP), the largest professional body that supports all practitioners, including students, nurses and ODPs, working with perioperative patients. The website (www.afpp.org.uk) offers educational materials, information, discussions and other resources.

Information about ODPs is available at www.aodp.org. The College of Operating Department Practitioners (CODP) supports the education of ODPs and has been instrumental in guiding the profession to develop to statutory registration.

Both of these websites hold valuable information which may help you to understand what to expect when you enter the doors of the operating department and meet your first perioperative patients. Other websites that may be of interest include www.proprius.org.uk (the Organization for Education, Training and Development Centres in Operating Department Practice) and www.aorn.org (website of the Association of Perioperative Registered Nurses).

If you want to undertake a general search of perioperative articles, try entering one of the following search terms in www.google.co.uk: 'perioperative care', 'theatre nursing', 'operating department practice', 'surgery' and 'anaesthesia'. More specialized articles about perioperative care can be found on PubMed: http://www.pubmedcentral.nih.gov/. A further reading list appears at the end of this section.

What your higher education institution can provide

Your higher education institution (HEI) may run perioperative courses and so you will have access to experts in perioperative care. If you know that you are going on a perioperative placement, or you are interested in doing so, you should contact your tutors and request lectures, sessions, clinical simulation of basic perioperative skills.

HEIs also often have clinical areas for simulated skills training. This can provide valuable experience of simulated perioperative experiences before working in the area. Skills training could include learning to scrub at real scrub sinks, learning to don gown and gloves, helping to drape patients, carrying out admission and discharge procedures and patient transfer.

You may find that your course of studies does not include a perioperative placement. If you are interested in visiting the area, you may wish to speak to your tutors to see whether they can organize a placement or a patient follow-through for you.

Challenges

The acute nature of the perioperative environment can provoke much anxiety in student nurses. This is a natural reaction to stress, and one of the many skills that you may learn in perioperative care is the ability to understand and manage your own reactions to stress.

Stressors in the perioperative environment include pressure to carry out activities rapidly, tense situations, interpersonal difficulties within the multidisciplinary team, confusion over role boundaries or requirements, and lack of knowledge or experience about situations. Stressful situations that can arise include:

• patients dying following unsuccessful surgery, adverse anaesthetic incidents or extensive trauma

- scrubbing for surgical procedures to help senior medical staff (you will normally scrub with a qualified practitioner, but you would still have responsibility to provide a high level of support to the surgeon)
- addressing ethical dilemmas such as whether to give a person who is dying and is a Jehovah Witness a blood transfusion
- organizing theatre lists
- managing conflicting situations, for example choosing when to send for the next patient while taking all factors into account
- identifying appropriate learning experiences and understanding when to ask for help, for example when a minor procedure goes wrong and becomes major (e.g. sudden haemorrhage, patient deterioration, complications developing or change in diagnosis mid-procedure)
- managing the theatre team and identifying priorities for patient care – senior nursing students are sometimes given the opportunity to manage appropriate theatre lists.

Conclusion

Caring for perioperative patients requires caring practitioners with knowledge and skills in delivering patient care in acute situations. A caring and skilled perioperative practitioner can mean the difference between an operation with poor patient outcomes and a stress-free surgical procedure that results in a satisfied, complication and pain-free patient. A career in perioperative care can be varied and interesting, allowing you to gain new knowledge and develop new skills in this rapidly developing area of patient care.

Further reading

Avidan M, Ginsburg R, Wendon J, Ponte J 2002 Perioperative care, anaesthesia, pain management and intensive care: an illustrated colour text. Churchill Livingstone, Edinburgh

Phillips N 2007 Berry & Kohn's operating room technique, 11th edn. Mosby, St Louis

Rothrock J 2006 Alexander's care of the patient in surgery. Mosby, St Louis

Wicker P, O'Neill J 2006 Caring for the perioperative patient (essential clinical skills). Blackwell, Oxford

Woodhead K, Wicker P 2005 A textbook of perioperative care. Elsevier, Edinburgh

6.13 Private hospital nursing

Anne Levington

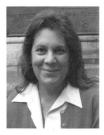

Practice Facilitator Independent Sector NHS,
Barts and the London Hospital,
London, UK

Over many years the independent sector has developed positive relationships and partnerships with the NHS in many areas of service delivery and commissioning. The independent, or private, sector comprises organizations that provide health care from non-public funding sources. They do not have the primary role of a 'teaching-focused delivery care system', as within the NHS.

Private hospital statuses are (profit or non-profit):

- charities
- multinational companies
- stand-alone clinics or surgeries
- care homes
- self-employed (independent practitioners).

The independent sector makes a vital contribution to the provision and delivery of health care in the UK, and to the economy. Independent healthcare providers work with a wide range of stakeholders, including patients and customers, consultants and their professional associations, regulatory bodies, intermediaries, the NHS and Primary Care Trusts, general practitioners and community health services.

Access to private health care is usually via:

- private healthcare insurance
- funded by the patient
- contractual agreement with a NHS organization.

Ensuring the quality of clinical care

All independent healthcare providers within the UK are regulated by the Department of Health inspectorates, such as the Healthcare Commission, and are inspected on a regular basis. Patients in the independent sector receive high standards of clinical care, and are treated in high-quality facilities.

One contribution from independent healthcare providers is in the area of education and facilitation of pre-registration student nurses and the overseas nurse programme. The majority of private hospitals in the UK have some form of affiliation with a higher educational institution, with the Independent Healthcare Advisory Services (2006) reporting that there are an estimated 6375 nurses employed in private hospitals, including a substantial number who are actively involved in providing nursing education and training in private hospitals. Private hospitals have continued to support and commit to training and education because of the associated positive outcomes. It is generally agreed that training and education improve the quality of health care. Other benefits include improvement of the work environment, recruitment and retention of staff.

Private hospitals in the UK have a strong commitment to the promotion of a culture that embraces professional development and a dedication to quality customer service inclusive of patients being informed and consulted about the nature of their treatment. In a private hospital, patients are empowered by having chosen not only their medical specialist but also the facility in which their treatment will be delivered. The private sector takes pride in providing the latest technology and an aesthetically pleasing environment.

Private hospitals within the UK are beginning to ensure that part of the students' 3-year programme will enable them to experience how health care is accessed within the private sector, and they are a viable alternative for students seeking clinical experiences. Learning opportunities similar to those offered in the public sector are available in most private hospitals.

Getting the most out of clinical placement at a private hospital

Preparation for your placement is the key, not only to greater understanding, but also to increased confidence in your clinical experience. Suggestions for preparation include:

- knowing what your educational institution's learning objectives are for your placement
- formulating your personal goals

- knowing what you need to do and see. If you are clear about what learning is required, you can maximize opportunities
- confirming shift times and rosters
- organizing transport and planning to arrive early or on time
- ensuring you have the appropriate uniform, including footwear and identification
- being interested and maximizing your learning opportunities.

Consider the following example.

Kate, a second-year nursing student was very excited about her clinical placement. She wanted to make a good first impression, so she contacted the mentor on her assigned ward and made arrangements to meet the mentor and orient herself to the ward before commencement. Such a strategy allowed Kate to be more at ease and familiar with the environment on her first day.

- Showing an interest in what is happening around you. Asking questions. Observing what the registered nurse does. Finding out what is happening and why. Researching and finding out more.

You will have many resources available to you, starting with experienced registered nurses and midwives. Practice facilitators or link lectures are also available in many areas. Some hospitals have library resources for your use, as well as access to research learning requirements.

Consider this example.

Amy, a third-year student, sought an opportunity to learn more about a procedure by arranging to observe the surgery being performed on her allocated patient. She initiated this learning experience herself, thus enhancing her understanding of her patient's condition and treatment, and taking responsibility for her learning.

Communication

- Talk to the nurses in your team. Voicing your needs will enable staff to assist you in reaching your expected learning outcomes. Expressing your knowledge of a situation will guide the nursing team in understanding your previous experiences and learning needs.

- Relating to the multidisciplinary team (doctors, physiotherapists, dieticians, etc.) can be quite daunting. Your clinical placement is a good opportunity to observe and learn how other nurses communicate in various situations.
- Effective communication is an essential nursing skill that you develop with experience. Use your clinical experience to improve how you communicate. Focus on developing professional relationships with the patients and their families. This will increase your confidence in caring for them. You will be more able to assess changes in their condition, and also offer comfort and understanding.

Using your initiative

- Within your set boundaries and competency of practice you have plenty of scope to use your initiative. It is important to recognize the difference between a patient's needs and wants, as this is imperative in deciding the priority of care. This is a vital component of critical thinking and decision-making.
- Your supernumerary status as a student nurse enables you to be part of the team but not part of the workforce. This will help your nursing team so that they then have the opportunity to show you a variety of specialized skills and enable you to follow your patient's journey from preoperative, perioperative and postoperative care during their stay in hospital.
- If you identify a patient need, follow through with action. If the action required is outside your scope of practice, a referral will be required. You can refer to your co-mentor, mentor, facilitator, and the ward sister or unit manager. The rewards of teamwork are so much more than sharing the physical loads. You will gain other benefits, as well as the gratitude of your co-workers — your self-worth and job satisfaction will soar.
- As student nurses will have experiences within NHS and private sector placements, they need to be fully aware that policies and procedures will be different, but the essence of the framework will be the same.
- All hospital policies and procedures should be readily available for your use in every clinical area. You are expected to adhere to these at all times. If you are unsure, ask your mentor or your facilitator.

The following is a scenario from a third-year student.

Ben was on clinical placement caring for a patient in a surgical unit. As the patient's doctor left the room, he asked Ben to remove the drain tube. Ben looked up the procedure in the policy and procedure manual, and was able to gather the necessary equipment. Ben's initiative ensured that he was confident to perform the procedure under the supervision of his grateful and impressed mentor.

Reference

Independent Healthcare Advisory Services 2006 2005 Credentials Document. Online. Available: http://www.independenthealthcare.org.uk/downloads/quality_initiatives/IHAS_2005_Credentials.pdf 28 Feb 2008

6.14 Public health and practice nursing

Elizabeth M. J. Porter

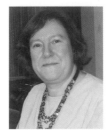

Programme Leader, School of Nursing and Midwifery,
University of Southampton,
Southampton, UK

Definition and overview of the practice nurse environment

Practice nurses are registered nurses who work in primary health care within a setting specific practice, usually a general practice. Practice nurses are normally employed by general practitioners (GPs) and work as part of a team of nurses who deliver nursing care to a practice population. The practice population can be defined as those individuals and their families who are registered with GPs within a GP practice. Practice nurses provide nursing care for the GP population where patients live or work or attend school. The main emphasis of their work is on the provision of comprehensive, coordinated and continuous services.

Public health in practice nursing can be described as the over-arching term for enabling activities that involve interactions around the health of the practice population. The public health aspect of this role involves the practice nurse in enabling people to achieve optimum health. This is undertaken through health surveillance, monitoring and evaluation of the health status of the practice population. This approach is a fundamental part of good practice, with the purpose of preventing disease and disability, promoting, protecting and maintaining health. In summary, the purpose of public health in practice nursing is to:

- improve the health and well-being of the practice population
- prevent disease and minimize its consequences
- prolong valued life
- reduce inequalities in health.

The importance of general practice as a learning experience

General practice is important as a learning experience for nursing students for a number of reasons.

Firstly, it provides them with contact with the practice population and the opportunity to deliver nursing care to people who may never access acute medical services provided by a hospital.

Secondly, it provides them with the opportunity to work alongside a practice nurse and their team, and to explore and apply essential nursing skills (Nursing and Midwifery Council 2006), and in particular the skills of public health nursing. Such an experience enables nursing students to question the perceived relationship between health, health care and disease, all of which have changed over time. This is evident in current calls for the National Health Service to become a 'health' not a 'sickness' service, to provide better prevention services with earlier intervention, to do more to tackle inequalities and to improve access to services (Department of Health 2006).

Finally, a general practice placement provides nursing students with the experience of participating in a range of public health activities carried out by the practice nurse and their team as part of targeting risk in the practice population, tackling inequalities in health and improving health in priority areas identified in National Service Frameworks (NSFs) (Porter 2005).

Learning opportunities available to nursing students in general practice

The public health learning opportunities available to nursing students can best be summarized in Table 6.1, which gives examples of practice nurse work developed around the ten National Occupational Standards for the practice of public health (Skills for Health 2004). The table also identifies a selection of the public health skills that nursing students will develop with the practice nurse team.

Relevant preparation for a learning placement in general practice

The demographics of a general practice population will have an impact upon the nature of public health activities in the practice.

Table 6.1   Ten occupational standards

Standard	Examples of public health activity in practice nursing	Skills required of practice nurses
Surveillance and assessment of the population's health and well-being	Profiling the practice population to identify those at risk of coronary heart disease or stroke Assessment of health needs Targeting individuals for screening or monitoring	The ability to: • collect, structure and read data • interpret, analyse and communicate information on health and well-being (health plans) • screen and monitor development through health • document evidence
Promoting and protecting the population's health and well-being	Promoting health: well women and men clinics addressing sexual health; contraception; menopause; osteoporosis; lifestyle factors such as diet, alcohol use, physical activity and smoking Protecting health: immunization for children, travellers and the elderly	The ability to: • develop, manage, implement and evaluate health promotion activity • teach, advise, facilitate and educate on health issues • implement infection control practices and Interpret codes of practice • immunize and vaccinate against disease
Developing quality and risk management within an evaluative culture	Developing and managing protocols for clinics Patient group directives for the administration of vaccines or drugs without prescription	The ability to: • manage medicines • use patient group directives • prescribe for children • work with risk management systems and evaluation strategies • maintain patient safety • deal with patient feedback and complaints • exercise clinical governance

table continues

Table 6.1   Ten occupational standards—Cont'd

Standard	Examples of public health activity in practice nursing	Skills required of practice nurses
Collaborative working for health and well-being	Teamwork with members of the general practice, health and social care professionals, and the voluntary sector within the local community, for example safeguarding children by using the Common Assessment Framework (CAF)	The ability to: • effectively lead, communicate (oral and written) and collaborate with others • motivate, raise consciousness and work with others • analyse, interpret and use information, self-appraisal and evaluation
Developing health programmes and services, and reducing inequalities	Development of a diabetes awareness event to improve diabetes care for the Asian practice populations	The ability to: • project plan, develop, implement, manage and evaluate
Policy and strategy development and implementation to improve health and well-being	Working with GPs to provide services in the general practice to meet recommendations of practice-based commissioning, for example developing a minor injuries clinic	The ability to: • appraise, audit, analyse, review, examine, promote • maintain awareness of social responsibility and change management • manage common minor injuries
Working with and for communities to improve health and well-being	Registration health checks for new members of the practice population Well-person checks, assessment of older people, dietary advice and monitoring, supporting patients with chronic disease	The ability to: • take a patient history, undertake physical assessment, identify and manage common medical conditions

table continues

Table 6.1 Ten occupational standards—Cont'd

Standard	Examples of public health activity in practice nursing	Skills required of practice nurses
Strategic leadership for health and well-being	Organization of practice nursing; management of the nurses' treatment room; nursing treatments and procedures; partnership working with practice population	The ability to: • organize, manage, think strategically and take appropriate action
Research and development to improve health and well-being	Providing evidence-based practice in delivery of nursing care, for example asthma management	The ability to: • evidence practice, critique evidence, implement and evaluate practice
Ethically managing self, people and resources to improve health and well-being	Working within the NMC code of professional conduct and protocols; policies and procedures laid down for the general practice	The ability to: • recognize caring as a moral imperative • take responsibility for self and actions

In preparation for your placement it is important to use the internet to access the world wide web (www) to identify the location of the general practice and its accessibility by public transport, and to search for information on the demography of the community local to the practice. Search the name of the Primary Care Trust (PCT) in which the general practice is situated, and look at the Director of Public Health's report on the state of health for that community. This will show you any specific health issues that it faces and you can then set learning outcomes for the placement that will enable you to build on your existing nursing skills.

Read sections of the 'Practice nurse handbook' (Hampson 2006) to familiarize yourself with the role of the practice nurse and reflect on your experiences as a user of the service offered by a general practice. Finally, contact the practice nurse team to determine start time and requirements of you for the placement visit.

Challenges that nursing students may encounter in general practice

Nursing students will learn how to apply nursing knowledge and skills within general practice, and to understand how and why this differs from nursing in the acute hospital sector. You will see quite different approaches to public health activity and how these improve health outcomes for the practice population, prevent hospital admissions and enable long-term conditions to be managed in the home. You will develop an understanding of how primary health care promotes health and provides treatments and care to the practice population and wider community.

Teamwork is paramount in general practice nursing. This means that you will need to understand the roles and responsibilities of the practice team, including the practice nurse, receptionist, practice manager, GP, medical secretary, paramedical staff and phlebotomist. These are the staff who are generally employed by the general practice, who are based in the general practice as either employees or partners of the GP(s).

It is also important for you to develop an awareness of the interface between general practice nurses and the wider community nursing team, and how multiagency and interprofessional working can benefit the practice population. To do this you need to understand the roles and responsibilities of:

- the members of the primary healthcare team (those employed by a PCT but working in partnership with general practice), including integrated nursing teams (district nurses, community staff nurses and healthcare assistants), specialist community public health nurses (health visitors and school nurses), midwives, community mental health nurses, community learning disability nurses and community matrons
- social services (employed by a local authority, unitary authority, borough or county), including social workers, home help and care workers
- voluntary services, including self-help groups and charities
- integrated health and social care teams, which include a mixture of all or some of the above and work in partnership to provide local communities with a more integrated health and social care service.

As a nursing student undertaking a practice placement you will have many experiences that will broaden your understanding of health care. Foremost among these will be the opportunity to witness practice nurses' roles in the commissioning process for the practice population – practice-based commissioning (PBC) (Department of Health 2005) – and how this improves the health of the community. You will also work with the practice nurse team in strategic planning of new services to meet the healthcare needs identified by the practice population, for example nurse-led services.

References

Department of Health 2005 Commissioning a patient-led NHS. HMSO, London

Department of Health 2006 Our health, our care, our say: a new direction for community services. HMSO, London

Hampson G 2006 Practice nurse handbook. Blackwell, Oxford

Nursing and Midwifery Council 2006 Essential skills clusters (ESCs). NMC Circular 35/2006. NMC, London

Porter E 2005 Public health in health visiting. In: Robotham A, Frost M (eds) Health visiting: specialist community public health nursing. Elsevier Churchill Livingstone, London, p 29–53

Skills for Health 2004 National occupational standards for practice of public health guide 2004. Skills for Health, Bristol. Online. Available at: http://www.skillsforhealth.org.uk 28 Feb 2008

6.15 Surgical nursing

Shoba Sookraj-Bahal

Lead Nurse for Pre-registration Education,
Homerton University Hospital NHS Foundation Trust,
London, UK

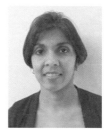

Surgical nursing is a specialist area of practice. Patients undergoing surgical interventions require a high standard of care and support from those in the healthcare profession who are responsible for their care. Knowledge and skills developed in this field of nursing are quite diverse and easily transferable. When caring for a surgical patient one needs to take a holistic approach, not only focusing on the surgery but also taking into consideration the physiological and psychological status of the patient both before and after surgery, as it is the individual patient's response to surgery, anaesthesia and intervention that determines the recovery period.

Surgical operations are classified into elective and emergency. With elective surgery, patients are seen in pre-assessment clinics before the operation and are therefore better prepared and perhaps less anxious, as opposed to emergency operations which must be done without delay.

Assessment is of paramount importance, both of the patient's understanding of the procedure and in detecting any potential post-operative complications that may have an impact on the patient's recovery. With the use of modern technology, such as keyhole surgery and less invasive procedures, the length of hospital stay has been greatly reduced. Monitoring the patient through the surgical experience involves early patient education so that patients can make informed choices and are less anxious. This leads to a seamless discharge and enhanced patient satisfaction.

Learning opportunities

Surgical nursing offers many exciting and educational opportunities for students. Not only will you explore the advances in surgical techniques and the effect these have on patients, you will also be able to understand how the anatomical structures were involved during surgery. It is therefore important to have a sound knowledge of human bioscience, which builds the platform for your clinical practice. You will also need to develop your observational and assessment skills to understand how to detect early signs of deterioration and how decisions are made concerning the care to be delivered. You will see several different venous access devices, including central lines and peripherally inserted intravenous lines as well infusion pumps and patient-controlled analgesia (PCA), and it will be important for you to know the purpose of these devices and how they work. You will also see a range of wounds and learn which type of dressing is appropriate, how they were closed (e.g. with sutures or staples). There will be opportunities to observe wound drainage systems that help to promote healing, and you will be taught the principles of monitoring and safe drain removal.

The surgical pace is quite fast and will prepare you to be a critical problem-solver, prioritizing your care efficiently and effectively, and ensuring that you make the appropriate clinical decisions. You will be encouraged to link patient diagnosis with the type of specialty surgery performed, and then relate this to the specifics of the patient. Only by obtaining a holistic approach will you be informed about the individual response to surgery. An excellent method of doing this is to follow the patient from the preoperative stage through to the intraoperative stage, then to the postoperative stage, and finally to the discharge stage. By following the patient's journey, you will be in a strong position to make the link between the patient and the operation. Questions that you could ask yourself during this experience include:

- Did the patient have any intraoperative complications?
- What measures were taken to prevent infection?
- What safety procedures were performed in the anaesthetic room?
- How was the patient's pain controlled?
- Were there any postoperative complications?

Preparing for the placement

Prior to your placement, some of your preparation should include revising the general principles of preoperative and postoperative care, including preoperative assessment, psychological preparation, physical assessment, informed consent, the importance of following specific postoperative instructions, the significance of monitoring your patient's vital signs, pain management, maintenance of fluid and electrolyte balance, maintenance of circulation, and prevention of postoperative complications (e.g. deep vein thrombosis and wound infection).

After establishing a general picture, move on to reviewing two or three surgical procedures for each specialty; for example, with orthopaedic surgery you may want to look at a hemiarthroplasty (knee replacement) and an arthroscopy. This is a useful exercise because, despite differences in surgery, there are generic principles that cross all specialties. You will also need to know the difference between septic and hypovolaemic shock, and their key indicators. It is important constantly to make references to each body system while learning about surgery. If a patient has a cholecystectomy, for example, you will need to understand exactly what the gallbladder does and what will happen if that organ is removed. In effect, your knowledge of body systems will be a vital resource, which you will constantly refer to during your surgical placement.

Surgical nursing is extremely rewarding and exciting, and will challenge and build upon your current knowledge and skills.

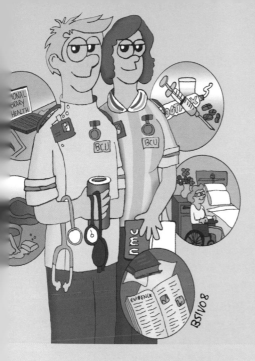

Glossary

Accountability
Relates to the forms of responsibility and duty, and to the notion of being responsible for your practice and potential consequences of any action or inaction.

Acculturation
The individual's adaptation to the customs, values, beliefs and behaviours of a new culture.

Acuity
The degree of complexity of a patient's state of illness and the level of care required.

Advocacy
A critical function of the nursing role that incorporates the ethical principle of beneficence, defending the rights of others or acting on their behalf.

Ageism
Prejudice against the older adult that perpetuates negative stereotyping of ageing as a period of decline.

Androgogy
The art and science of helping adults learn; a term coined by Malcolm Knowles to describe his theory of adult learning.

Assess
To gather, summarize and interpret relevant data about a learner or patient to make a decision or plan.

Best practice
The use of high-quality clinical evidence to inform and underpin patient care decisions and nursing actions.

Clinical governance
A framework designed to help nurses continuously to improve quality and to safeguard standards of practice. Clinical governance management encourages openness about strengths and weaknesses, and incorporates the need to be pro-active through best practice to promote excellence in health care and through lifelong learning.

Clinical learning environment
The placement location in a healthcare facility where nursing students are allocated in order to achieve objectives, care for clients/patients and undertake assigned learning activities.

Competence
Competence represents the overall ability of an individual to perform effectively within a role. This includes the knowledge, skills, attitudes and experience to undertake a whole role to the standard expected of like persons within a similar environment.

Compliance
Willingness to accept or follow treatment or regimens or practices prescribed or established by others.

Confidentiality
A binding social contract or covenant; a professional obligation to respect privileged information between health provider and client, and between staff and students.

Culturally competent health care
The ability to demonstrate sensitivity, knowledge and understanding of another person's culture, and to accept and respect cultural differences by adapting interventions to be congruent with those of that specific culture when delivering health care.

Culture
A complex concept that is an integral part of each person's life. It includes knowledge, beliefs, values, morals, customs, traditions and habits acquired by the members of a society.

Disability
A difficulty or inability to perform some key functions of living.

Duty
Responsibility; professional expectation.

Educational institution
An institution, such as a university, that provides an accredited nursing programme.

Ethical dilemma
A problem in which there is a moral or ethical choice to be made between choices that seem equally unfavourable.

Ethics
Guiding principles of human behaviour; morals.

Ethnicity
A dynamic and complex concept referring to how members of a group perceive themselves and how, in turn, they are perceived by others in relation to the population subgroup's common heritage of customs, characteristics, language and history.

Ethnocentrism
Belief that one's own culture is superior and that all other cultures are less sophisticated.

Feedback
Valid and reliable judgements about students' performance for the purposes of recognizing strengths and areas for improvement. Feedback provides students with information about what they are expected to do and how they are progressing. Ideally it is provided about all activities or situations in which the student has been involved.

Healthcare facility
An institution where the delivery of health care is the primary focus. Examples include hospitals, outpatient clinics, medical centres and nursing homes. These may be publicly or privately operated.

Healthcare team
A multidisciplinary group of healthcare professionals and non-professionals who provide services to patients and their families in an attempt to maximize the optimal health and well-being of the person to whom their activities are directed.

Horizontal violence
Covert or overt dissatisfaction directed by nurses towards one another and towards those less powerful than themselves. Usually it is nurses in the least organizationally powerful positions that manifest bullying among themselves and towards those with even less power.

Learning environment facilitator (or practice education facilitator)
Registered nurses who are based in National Health Service Trusts and the independent sector to support mentors and manage practice-based learning issues.

Learning objectives
The outcomes or goals that students wish to achieve, agreed in negotiation with mentors while in the clinical placement.

Link lecturer
Responsible for liaising with clinical staff to monitor the quality of practice experiences; offers support to students and registered nurses.

Multidisciplinary healthcare team
The different disciplinary groups of people responsible for working as a team to provide high-quality health care to patients.

Mentor
Nurse who supports a nursing student during practice experience; takes responsibility for supervising, directly or indirectly, the student's practice.

National Health Service (NHS)
UK system of public health care.

Negligence
A failure to provide a degree of care expected of you, in the eyes of the law, resulting in loss or injury to an individual.

Nursing and Midwifery Council (NMC)
Regulatory body for nurses and midwives in the UK (previously United Kingdom Central Council for Nursing, Midwifery and Health Visiting, UKCC).

Patient-centred care
A way of practising that focuses on an individual's personal beliefs, values, wants, needs and desires. An approach in which patients' freedom to make their own decisions is recognized as a fundamental and valuable human right.

Practice proficiency
A student is deemed proficient when they have successfully met all the NMC standards of proficiency for nursing, midwifery or specialist community public health nursing, or the relevant outcomes of an NMC specialist practice qualification, at the end of an NMC-approved programme. Practice proficiency may be signed off only by a practice teacher or a mentor who has met the additional NMC criteria.

Practice teacher
A registered nurse who has gained knowledge, skills and competence in both their specialist area of practice and in their teaching role; facilitates student learning, supervises and assesses students in the practice setting; and has undertaken an NMC-approved teacher preparation programme, or equivalent, and successfully achieved the outcomes defined in stage 4 of the developmental framework.

Primary Care Trust (PCT)
A component of the NHS. These Trusts are responsible for assessing the health needs of the population in a specified region and commissioning services to meet those needs.

Privacy
Protecting the patient from public view to promote dignity in caring or sensitive situations. A right for all individuals that protects their personal information and the dissemination of such information.

Reflection
A process by which nurses explore their clinical experience and their understanding of what they are doing and why they are doing it, and consider the impact it has on themselves and others.

Reflection promotes learning from practice by exploring, questioning and growing through, and as a consequence of, clinical experiences.

Registered nurse
A person who is registered to practise nursing in the UK and whose name is recorded on the Nursing and Midwifery Council (NMC) register.

Sexual harassment
Conduct of a sexual nature that is unwanted and unwelcome by the receiver. Conduct is considered unwelcome when it is neither invited nor solicited, and the behaviour is deemed offensive and undesirable.

Sign-off mentor
A suitably qualified mentor who is able to sign off students' final practice placement.

Index